DASH DIET FOR BEGINNERS

28-DAY LOW SODIUM MEAL PLAN FOR A HEALTHY EATING LIFESTYLE WITH 50 SAVORY RECIPES

NOOK AND NOURISH

ISBN: 979-8-9863147-0-9

Disclaimer

This book is presented to you for informational purposes only and is not a substitute for any kind of professional, medical/health advice. The content of this book is based solely on the personal views and opinions of the author, should not be considered scientific or correct conclusions, and do not represent the views of others. All information presented here is "as is" and without warranty of any kind, expressed or implied. Although we strive to provide accurate general information in this book, we do not guarantee that the content is free from errors or omissions, and you should not rely solely on this information. Always consult a professional in the area for your particular needs and circumstances before you make any professional, business, legal, and financial or tax-related decisions. The author of this book does not render any professional advice. You agree that under no circumstances, will the author and/or our officers, employees, successors, shareholders, joint venture partners or anyone else working with the author be liable for any direct, indirect, incidental, consequential, equitable, special, punitive, exemplary or any other damages resulting from your use of this book including but not limited to all the content, information, stories and products presented here.

We may share success stories of other people in this book as examples to motivate you, but it does not serve as a guarantee or promise of any kind for your results and successes if you decide to use the information and medical/health tips offered here. It is your sole responsibility to independently review the content presented here and any decisions you make and the consequences thereof are your own. We reserve the right to update the content and information in this book from time to time as needed.

CONTENTS

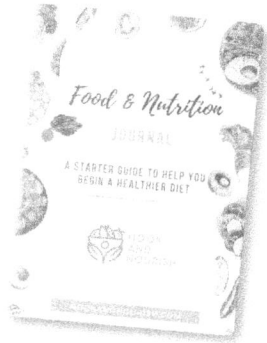

Congratulations on pursuing your journey to creating a healthy eating lifestyle with the DASH Diet! We wanted to give you extra tools to help you on this new crusade.
If you'd like more free recipes, a free printable food journal to track your meals, and a nutritional calculator please visit; www.nookandnourish.com or scan the QR code below.

~ Nook and Nourish

INTRODUCTION

Between the stress of success and the agony of defeat, sitting with the fans during a football game is enough to raise your blood pressure. It's not just the 120 decibels of cheering that lure you to gorge; there are also the greasy hot dogs and salty chips.

The ancient Greeks would have had a very different experience at games than we do today, as they had a healthy eating culture. They ate lots of fresh vegetables and fruits, nuts, beans and legumes, wheat bread, olive oil, and rarely meat or dairy products.

Have you heard of the DASH Diet?

The DASH Diet is a nutritional plan that emphasizes eating many fruits, vegetables, and whole grains while limiting your intake of fat, salt, and sugar. It is a plan for lowering hypertension and reducing the overall risk of heart disease and diabetes.

You may wonder, how the DASH Diet is good for people with diabetes. This is not a diet that will cure your diabetes. However, it could help control your blood sugar levels, keeping them in a manageable range.

Do you want to start a low-sodium diet and still enjoy the foods that you like? If so, then this diet is for you. The DASH Diet is a great low-sodium diet and it can help you eat the foods that you love while still reducing your sodium intake to very low levels.

Maybe you're tired of trying different diets, exercising, and still not getting the results that you want. This diet is very effective in helping people to lose weight, lower cholesterol, lower blood pressure and even control their blood sugar levels.

The DASH Diet is one of the most popular diets in the world today. This plan has helped millions of Americans improve their cardiovascular health through foods that are nutritionally dense with healthy fats, carbohydrates, and proteins.

I have been a victim of hypertension and high blood pressure for the past seventeen years and, as the founder of Nook and Nourish, I would like to share my knowledge about the DASH Diet with you. It has been a game-changer for me. It has helped to lower my blood pressure and cholesterol levels and improved my heart health.

Helping you reduce your hypertension levels and risk of diabetes matters to me. I am here to provide you with the tools that will help you on your health improvement journey.

This book approaches the diet plan from the perspective of enjoying the foods that you love while lowering your hypertension and blood sugar levels to live a happier and more fulfilled life. It will encourage victims of hypertension and diabetes to stick with a meal plan not just until their symptoms subside, but for their entire life journey.

We'll cover common DASH Diet questions and address health concerns, compare other diets, and provide a printable food journal, so you get a better understanding of what you eat on a daily and weekly basis.

Written in an easy-to-understand language, this 28-day action plan is packed with information that will help you implement this diet plan in your everyday life.

Great recipes for diets like these are sometimes hard to find. I have included fifty delicious recipes in this book, and you will easily find all the ingredients at your local grocery store. I've also added dairy alternatives for our lactose-intolerant friends. So make sure that you take the time to review them and then get cooking!

I urge you to get out there and start using the DASH Diet plan. The benefits that you'll receive from one of the best diets around will surprise you.

Some may call this a labor of love, but this book represents my journey toward good health. I want to share with you all that I have learned about this plan. Enough with failing diets, expensive gym memberships, and endless exercise programs! It's time to clean up your diet, start eating a low-sodium meal plan and prioritize your health. Get out of your comforter and get excited about living a healthier lifestyle. Who knows? You might fall in love with the diet plan so much that you'll consider making it a lifestyle habit. Start thinking about what your body needs to get healthy and enjoy the food you love.

1

WHAT IS THIS THING CALLED THE DASH DIET?

Endorsed by the United States National Heart, Lung, and Blood Institute, the DASH (Dietary Approaches to Stop Hypertension) Diet studies the nutrient composition of food items to prepare unique dietary strategies that help to reduce high blood pressure. The diet is a result of the engineering done by biologists and lawmakers on a quest to find what components to eliminate from one's diet to control rising blood pressure.

The DASH Diet came about because of the rising number of people with high blood pressure. The number has almost doubled in the last two decades. This led medical experts, along with the United States Department of Health and Human Services, to look for ways to deal with hypertension and eliminate the risks associated with high blood pressure. After a careful study, researchers found that people who consumed more vegetables or who followed a plant-based diet showed fewer signs of rising blood pressure. This, therefore, became the foundation of the DASH Diet.

Using the DASH Diet, people focus on eating organic foods rather than processed foods. Whole grains, fruit, vegetables, and lean meats form the essential components of this diet plan. In extreme cases, people with major signs of heart-related ailments caused by high blood pressure are also advised to go vegan for a while to lower hypertension.

This nutritional plan also sets out strict guidelines for salt consumption. Because too much salt and oil significantly raise the blood pressure in the human body, the DASH Diet guidelines significantly reduce the salt intake. The recipes that follow this diet include a wholesome mix of green vegetables, natural fruit, low-fat dairy products, and lean protein such as chicken, fish, and plenty of beans. Besides limiting the intake of salt, the rule of thumb is to minimize food items rich in red meat, processed sugars, and composite fat. Per standard practice, anyone following the DASH Diet is advised not to consume more than one teaspoon (2,300 mg) of sodium a day.

This diet is safe and accredited by the United States Department of Agriculture (USDA). The US Dietary Guidelines also included the DASH Diet as one of three healthy diets recommended between 2015 and 2020.

IS IT EFFECTIVE FOR EVERYONE?

Although DASH Diet studies show that low salt intake results in the biggest reduction in blood pressure, the effects of salt restriction on longevity and health are not well established.

When a person has high blood pressure, reducing salt consumption has a significant impact on their blood pressure. However, salt reduction has a much smaller effect on people with normal blood pressure. Salt sensitivity—meaning salt increases blood pressure more for some people—may be responsible for this. The DASH Diet is an excellent option for anyone wanting to keep their heart healthy. This diet is recommended if you have:

- Chronic Kidney Disease (CKD)—People with CKD are advised to get their kidneys checked and follow a strict DASH Diet. Because they have an increased risk of dehydration and cardiovascular disease, a higher salt intake can put them at risk of further damaging their kidneys. CKD is a condition that occurs as a result of gradual kidney damage. This leads the body to produce less urine. A person with CKD can no longer rid their bodies of harmful waste or toxins. The DASH Diet reduces salt intake along with a variety of unhealthy foods, which helps people with CKD to improve their overall health and relieve the condition. A study by The National Kidney

Foundation of the United States found that the DASH Diet decreases blood pressure; lowers the risk of heart disease, cancer, and stroke; and reduces the chance of kidney stone development.

- Hypertension—People who have been diagnosed with hypertension have a high chance of developing heart-related illnesses. Hypertension occurs when the blood pressure levels in your body increase beyond normal levels. It is one of the primary causes of heart attacks and strokes. However, with a strict DASH Diet and exercise, people suffering from hypertension can lower their blood pressure by over 10 percent. According to the American Heart Association, the DASH Diet can lower blood pressure in as little as two weeks.

Studies show that in addition to other comprehensive care, this diet can help to reduce insulin sensitivity, inflammation, and cholesterol. This helps to control the effects of diabetes mellitus and metabolic syndrome.

You don't have to have a preexisting condition to go on the DASH Diet. It is also suitable for the general population. The diet is not considered a cure for hypertension.

One of the key factors with any dieting plan is consistency. Following a healthy diet that you can actually stick to is essential. There is no dieting plan in the world that will work for everyone since all of us are unique. With that in mind, the DASH Diet was designed to reduce blood pressure, and it can accomplish that goal. Still, that won't do you any good if you don't follow through.

The greatest reduction in blood pressure is experienced by those who follow the low-sodium version of the plan. This should come as no surprise since a reduction in salt intake has been shown to significantly reduce blood pressure.

My point here is that lowering your salt intake while changing to whole foods is a much healthier choice, but you must ensure that any dieting plan is suited to your personal taste.

THE HISTORY AND BACKGROUND OF THE DASH DIET

This diet was developed in the 1990s. The National Institute of Health (NIH) funded research projects to develop dietary interventions that could help control the rising hypertension issue.

According to the National Institute of Health, dietary approaches were particularly helpful for the maintenance of blood pressure in patients, with and without hypertension. Dr. Walter Willett of Harvard University, Dr. Eric Rimm of Tufts University, and Dr. Frank Hu and his team in China were all awarded grants from the NIH to create tailored food approaches for lowering high blood pressure.

In the United States, one out of every four people has been diagnosed with hypertension. Hypertension is a silent killer because there are no symptoms. High blood pressure can kill you silently from the inside. There were many medicinal solutions to alleviate high blood pressure. Yet, scientists have struggled to find a consistent and harmless solution for patients.

Scientists have made many modifications during experiments. Hypertension raises the risk of heart disease with an estimated 2,000 people dying of heart disease in the United States every day.

The DASH Diet originated in 1997 as a randomized, controlled feeding study. The original researchers found that it improved systolic and diastolic blood pressure across genders, races, and in those with pre-hypertension and hypertension. Since the results of the original study were published, the DASH Diet has formed a key component of national guidelines on blood pressure.

However, national adherence to the DASH Diet is very low. There are many reasons for this, including food deserts, the prevalence of nutrient-dense food, and the cost of the diet. *Food deserts* are areas without access to fresh fruit and vegetables and where education levels are low. The DASH Diet is a whole food, plant-based diet that does not contain processed or fast foods, such as chips, candies, soda, and fried foods. The US Dietary Guidelines recommend a healthy balanced diet for everyone. They do not recommend changing any food groups that have been found to be effective in lowering blood pressure.

The original study included 459 participants with stage 1 hypertension. All participant food was provided. The control group ate the Standard American Diet, with emphasis on refined grains, dairy fats, meat, and sugar; and little fruit, vegetables, and nuts. The experimental group was placed on the DASH Diet, which contained fruit, vegetables, fat-free and low-fat dairy products, whole grains, fish, and poultry.

The study found that about half of the stage 1 hypertension patients lowered their blood pressure with the DASH Diet. Blood pressure dropped by 11 points for those in the first hypertensive stage, and 12 points for those with pre-hypertension. The DASH Diet lowered systolic blood pressure by 7.5 points and diastolic blood pressure by 4.1 points.

While the DASH Diet was effective for hypertension patients, not many people adhered to it after the study ended. The reasons may have been nutritional restrictions. Nonetheless, the study helped to prove that a balanced diet with reduced sodium and lower saturated fat, can decrease blood pressure and protect against stroke and heart disease.

HOW THE DASH DIET WORKS

As this diet gained popularity, experts began studying the effectiveness of the plan. New research showed that the DASH plan lowered blood pressure in just two weeks. In multiple studies, people who experienced the best results on the plan (meaning a significant decline in blood pressure after just fourteen days) had moderately high blood pressure or pre-hypertension before starting the plan. The DASH Diet helped to improve medication response even in people with severe hypertension who couldn't eliminate their blood pressure medication during the studies. Additional research demonstrated that this nutritional plan is the safest weight loss diet for adults and teens and that it helps with cognitive function, decreases the incidence of kidney stones, and protects against certain types of cancers and chronic health conditions. It also helps to reduce the incidence of stroke and osteoporosis, and insulin resistance in type 2 diabetes. Bottom line: the research supports the claim that the DASH Diet encourages optimal body function.

Doctors and nutritionists thoughtfully constructed this diet plan to provide liberal amounts of nutrients critical for optimal body function. *Improved function* means better internal communication so that each bodily system works properly and is well connected to other systems. This improved function and communication promotes healthy cardiovascular (heart) and gastrointestinal (digestion) systems and leads to better overall weight management.

These critical nutrients are found in natural food, which sounds simple enough. However, many diets promote the use of processed foods, which not only lack vital nutrients but contain numerous artificial components that the body can't easily break down and process. The real-food crux of the DASH Diet is a very different, yet simple, approach: an eating plan that is rich in vegetables and fruits, 100 percent whole grains, beans, lean meats, and low-fat and nonfat dairy products. These natural foods have been designed by nature to nourish and optimally fuel the body.

This is where the DASH Diet differs: It doesn't make promises. It's not even really a diet. The word *diet* has come to indicate some significant temporary change in eating habits to achieve some physical change, at which point the diet is over. This nutritional plan is the complete opposite: a long-term approach to eating as a commitment to health. It is an eating plan designed to promote and support healthy lifestyle changes, making weight loss a lovely by-product of the plan! Healthy "real food" guidelines and eating plans allow individuals and entire families to commit to a realistic way of living and eating as a part of daily life. By equipping the body with the right foods to fight off chronic disease and weight gain, the DASH Diet helps people achieve excellent health.

This diet will help you change your eating habits with little effort and no guesswork. Implementing it is easy, and it's likely to be a well-received change in your lifestyle. Moreover, it can be continued for life! The plan is designed to improve your long-term health.

1. **Eat natural, unprocessed foods like fruits, vegetables, whole grains, and nuts.** It is all about returning to natural, unprocessed foods that have always been part of the human diet. Nature has designed these foods to nourish and optimally fuel our bodies.

2. **Make olive oil your primary source of dietary fat.** Fat is so important to the human diet, but this plan calls for a reduction in the consumption of animal products and unhealthy fats. "Animal fats are high in simple and saturated fats," said Dr. Ron Rosedale, former director of the Cardiac Center at Banner Good Samaritan Medical Center and author of *The Rosedale Diet Book*. We should consume only essential fatty acids (good fats) like those found in EVOO, fish oil, flaxseed oil, avocado oil, nuts, and seeds. These are truly extraordinary foods.

3. **Reduce your consumption of red meat.** Red meats, such as beef, lamb, and pork, all contain high levels of saturated fat. A study by the American Institute of Medicine found an association between the regular consumption of red meat with a higher risk of heart disease.

4. **Eat limited amounts of fish and white meat.** Fish, like salmon and tuna, contains high levels of beneficial omega-3 fatty acids DHA and EPA. Researchers have found that these fatty acids dilate

blood vessels, lower triglycerides (blood fats), and lower the risk of heart disease.

Depending on your reasons for embarking on this diet, there may be various effects and outcomes. According to the American Heart Association, the DASH Diet can help "prevent or postpone CKD events and target specific risk factors including elevated blood pressure, lipids (cholesterol and triglycerides), insulin resistance, and arterial stiffness." It can also:

- Lower your intake of sodium. This, in conjunction with a higher intake of calcium, magnesium, and potassium, works to lower overall blood pressure due to the biological functions each mineral plays. For example, homeostasis between sodium and potassium is a key component in blood pressure and the renin-angiotensin-aldosterone (RAAS) system. *The RAAS system* is an important part of the body's blood pressure regulation and the entire process of regulating the cardiovascular system. The human body needs calcium to maintain smooth muscle tone (smooth muscle regulates blood vessel tone), magnesium is necessary for the proper function of the muscles that control blood flow, and sodium activates the RAAS system. The DASH Diet increases the consumption of these minerals and, thus, helps to control blood pressure levels.

- Reduce your risk of hypertension. Hypertension is a major risk factor for cardiovascular disease and is a comorbid (the simultaneous presence of two or more diseases) condition common with type 2 diabetes and obesity it's also a risk factor for CKD. There are two types of hypertension: preexisting and reactive. Preexisting hypertension refers to individuals who have high blood pressure at the time of the test, while reactive hypertension is characterized by a sudden, extreme elevation in blood pressure caused by a triggering stressor. Individuals suffering from reactive hypertension tend to have higher levels of stress and anxiety, lower social support, and an increased frequency of negative life events. Most commonly, this type of hypertension is brought on by a life event like a death or business failure. In general, reactive hypertension is more common and affects 25–50 percent of individuals with preexisting hypertension.
- In addition, some studies have found that the DASH Diet can reduce the risk of developing type 2 diabetes. This population has an elevated risk for CKD: 60 percent for non-white men and 40 percent for both black and white women.
- Aid with weight loss. "Weight loss on a DASH Diet is most commonly achieved by a caloric restriction," says Dr. Rosedale. This is accomplished by eating foods high in fiber—such as the fruit and vegetables

that are part of this nutritional plan—and avoiding foods that contain added sugars, saturated fats and sodium.

WHAT CAN YOU EXPECT FROM THIS DIET?

Unhealthy eating habits have played a major role in the decline of many people's health, paving the way for the introduction of numerous diet plans. Some of them worked, while others didn't, but the DASH Diet has proven to be a successful approach for many people.

This diet can help you to lose weight and improve your health at the same time. What's more amazing about this diet is that it does not demand very strict rules. The DASH Diet is realistic, focusing on decreasing overall calorie intake while increasing your intake of necessary nutrients.

You will quickly feel better when you start following this nutritional plan. Prepare for this diet according to your life-style and needs. Avoid eating junk food before starting, as junk food contains unhealthy fats and sugars which can hamper your weight loss efforts.

You will consume more fiber than you do on a regular basis, and this may not be possible if your regular diet is full of high levels of saturated fats and sugars. Along with increasing your intake of fresh fruit and vegetables, you may have to change your cooking methods. This means that you must stop deep-frying your food and begin cooking more on the grill or stovetop.

If you suffer from high cholesterol, it is important that you change your diet. Changing the way you eat can definitely help to lower your cholesterol and improve your overall heart health but it is not a permanent solution to the problem.

The DASH Diet is meant to be a long-term health commitment and dietary eating pattern. Depending on the starting point, individuals will have to make several changes to their current diet. People who suffer from hypertension may have to start by changing only a few aspects of their diet. Though for many people this diet will be just what they needed.

Do not expect this diet to be a short-term fix. Many people do not sustain their health benefits over an extended period of time — even if they're following all the dietary recommendations to the letter. This is because it takes time for your body to adjust and realize the benefits of eating such a low-sodium diet. To achieve the most benefits and the longest-lasting health gains, individuals must devote themselves to the nutritional plan.

HOW TO START YOUR DIET

The DASH eating plan is simple to follow. Even tiny modifications made over time can have a big impact. Follow these steps to start living a healthy lifestyle for the rest of your life:

1. Assess Your Current State

It is important to track and monitor your current daily intake of nutrients. This includes your consumption of all food categories, including fruit, fat, meat, grain, and dairy products. Start writing a daily list of your meals and snacks. Remember to be as accurate as possible with the amount of food you consume. This eating plan does not require any particular foods or recipes that are difficult to follow. Make notes about the frequency of your consumption of various food groups so that you can keep track of them over time. Visit our website at www.nookandnourish.com for your free printable food journal.

Make use of a free, interactive, online Body Weight Planner to find out how many calories you should consume to lose weight. This online tool is useful for estimating how many calories your body needs on a daily basis and is a good guide for the DASH nutritional plan.

2. Seek Your Doctor's Advice on Your Medication

Before starting a diet, it is important to look into the potential effects of your current medication. If you are currently taking medications, ask your doctor whether there are any possible interactions between your medications and the DASH Diet. You do not need to modify your current medication for this diet. It is recommended that you inform your doctor about any dietary changes that you decide to make.

This is especially the case when you are already on hypertension medication. In this case, you must talk to your doctor before stopping the medication, and ask about any possible side effects related to stopping the drug and starting a new diet plan.

3. Introduce the DASH Diet to Your Lifestyle

If you are going to adopt a new diet plan, then you will need some time and will have to apply some effort. This diet is simple, and you can easily incorporate it into your daily eating habits—all without making too many changes or sacrifices.

Adhere to crucial lifestyle recommendations, such as maintaining a healthy weight, engaging in regular physical activity, and drinking alcohol in moderation. This will help ensure that your body adapts to the changes you're making and that you will reap the health benefits of following the DASH Diet.

4. Make the DASH Diet a Family Affair

This eating plan can be a lifestyle change for the whole family. Start by changing your own food habits. It will help your children become accustomed to the diet. If you and your children have unhealthy eating habits, they are likely to follow suit.

Your family's support is important if you are to successfully apply the DASH Diet. Partner with your family to make healthy lifestyle changes that will have a positive impact on your overall health and well-being.

5. Don't Be Alarmed

At times, it may feel like you're not getting the right nutrients and balance of foods. Still, many users report feeling better than ever on the DASH Diet, even after just a few days. Making a lifestyle change is not easy, but it's easier for some than others. Some of the changes made may feel like sacrifices that you have to overcome. Look for helpful tips and tricks or motivational videos to remain positive when the time comes to change your eating habits. Some people find that seeing a positive result after only a week is enough to keep them going.

2

THE DASH VS. THE REST

I know you are probably wondering: Just how well does the DASH Diet compare to other diets? I can't tell you for sure, but I have been able to get enough data to compare the DASH Diet with other dietary plans.

By comparing this nutritional plan with other popular diets, you can see that the DASH plan is far more flexible and forgiving than the others. Any individual can follow it — even those who are obese. You don't have to make drastic dietary changes when you choose this diet.

I will compare the DASH Diet with the following popular diets:

1. The Mediterranean Diet
2. The Keto Diet

3. The Paleo Diet

Because of its high protein and low sugar content, the DASH Diet is similar to these popular diets. It's also low in fat and high in fiber, both of which are essential for maintaining a healthy metabolism. It is, however, the only mainstream diet that focuses on lowering salt levels. In many ways, the DASH Diet varies from the other dietary plans. The first way is the fact that it is not a "diet" per se, but more of a lifestyle change that still allows you to enjoy delicious foods.

Without further ado, let's take a look at the main similarities and differences between the DASH Diet and other diets:

1. **General Nutrition:** All of these diets strongly emphasize eating a variety of nutritious foods and reducing or eliminating foods that can harm your health. They all discourage eating highly processed foods commonly found in most modern diets. The concept that a diet rich in fruit and vegetables, nuts, legumes, whole grains, and healthy fats can promote excellent health is central to all of these diets. However, the DASH Diet has more specific guidelines than the other plans, guiding users to eat foods that are low in sodium, high in potassium and calcium, and a combination of polyunsaturated and monounsaturated fats.
2. **Health Benefits:** The DASH Diet has been widely researched and it's been demonstrated to lower

blood pressure in both hypertensive and non-hypertensive people. It has also been shown to decrease the risk of cardiovascular disease, heart disease, and stroke. This diet has proven to be a better dietary approach than others because it dilutes sodium intake by one gram per day. As a matter of fact, a study published in the *New England Journal of Medicine* showed that a DASH Diet can reduce blood pressure by up to 8 points.

3. **Weight Loss:** While the DASH Diet allows you to follow a lower-calorie target plan, it may not help you lose weight as easily as other popular diets. It's critical to stick to the DASH Diet if you want to lose weight. According to research, participants who followed the DASH nutritional plan lost more weight than those who didn't. The key is sticking to the diet for the long term. The DASH Diet does not have a rapid weight loss phase or a specific weight loss goal. Rather, it is a nutritious diet that emphasizes the consumption of fresh fruit and vegetables, lean meat, and low-fat dairy products.

4. **Sustainability:** The DASH Diet may be more difficult to follow than other diets. It necessitates a reduction in overall salt consumption. It remains a low-sodium diet even if you don't go out of your way to cut back on sodium. If you are not used to consuming so little salt, you should make a lifestyle modification. Unlike many fad diets based on one-

week results, you may have to make gradual changes as you progress with the DASH Diet. You will have to make small adjustments in your normal eating habits and drop foods that are not beneficial. With that said, if you follow the DASH Diet faithfully, it will provide you with all the health benefits you need. Your body will have more than enough sodium and other vitamins and minerals to function properly.

A typical serving guide (2000-calorie diet) for a patient following the DASH nutritional plan is as follows:

- **Vegetables:** 3-5 servings per day

  o *Single Serving Example: 1 cup raw spinach*

- **Fruit:** 3-5 servings per day

  o *Single Serving Example: 1/4 cup raisins*

- **Dairy foods:** two and a half servings per day
- **Lean meat, fish or poultry:** six ounces (about 40–50 grams) per day
- **Nuts and seeds:** one ounce (30 grams) per day
- **Eggs:** one per day
- **Low-fat or fat-free milk:** 1-2 servings per day
- **Fats and oils:** Limit to 6–9 teaspoons of oil per day

- **Grains:** 6 to 8 servings per day

    o *Single Serving Example:* 1/2 cup whole grain rice or barley

- **Beverages (excluding water):** two cups of coffee, tea, or hot chocolate; limit alcoholic beverages to one drink per day.

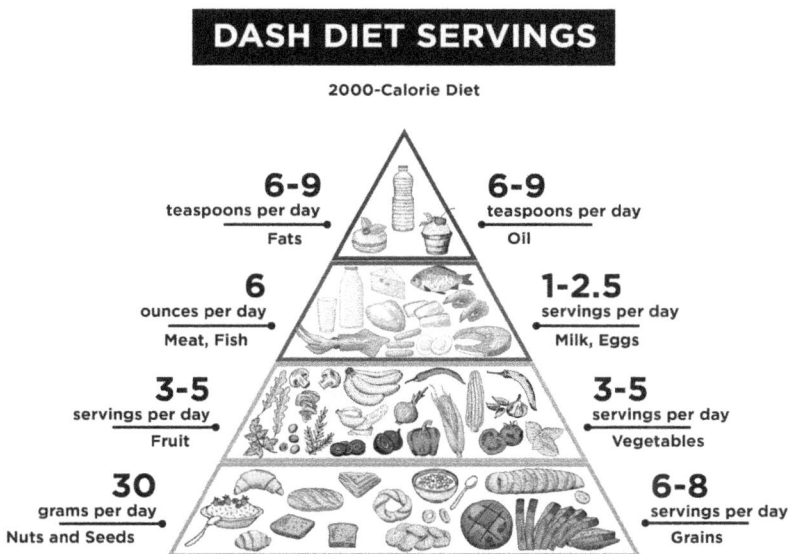

DASH DIET SERVINGS

2000-Calorie Diet

6-9 teaspoons per day — Fats

6-9 teaspoons per day — Oil

6 ounces per day — Meat, Fish

1-2.5 servings per day — Milk, Eggs

3-5 servings per day — Fruit

3-5 servings per day — Vegetables

30 grams per day — Nuts and Seeds

6-8 servings per day — Grains

Next, we'll take a closer look at these recommendations.

CARBOHYDRATES

Carbohydrates should account for 40 to 50 percent of your total calories, with added sugars or sweeteners accounting for no more than 10 percent of that. The exact percentage varies depending on how much exercise you get, but it is normally around 40 percent.

Instead of processed grains, choose whole grains like oatmeal, brown rice, barley, whole wheat bread, and brown pasta. Although whole grains include more vitamins and minerals than refined grains, high-fiber fruits, vegetables, and legumes appear to be better for your health.

A high-carbohydrate diet is not recommended. Instead of processed carbs like sugar, white bread, and cakes, the DASH Diet recommends that you consume whole-grain items. When it comes to carbs, this nutritional plan recommends high-fiber meals that include fruit, vegetables, and legumes. The intake of dried beans, peas, and lentils to increase your fiber intake while keeping your overall carbohydrate consumption low is also recommended.

FATS

Reduce the amount of fats you consume on a daily basis. Although some experts believe you should consume less, the total amount of fat in your diet should not exceed 35 percent of your entire daily calorie intake.

The DASH Diet plan is a low-fat diet because it limits the amount of saturated fat and trans fat in the diet. These fats are not good for your heart health. The DASH nutritional plan recommends that you consume no more than 5 percent saturated and trans fats of the recommended daily total fat consumption.

Plant-based fat sources include avocados and avocado oil, nuts, seeds, and olive oil. Animal products are a major source of saturated and trans fat in the diet. Red meat and processed meat, such as bacon, can contain up to 32 percent saturated fat. Dairy products such as milk or cheese may contain up to 14 percent saturated fat. Other animal products that can contain more than 10 percent saturated fat include duck and goose.

A research review published in *The American Journal of Clinical Nutrition* in 2010 showed that people who consumed a diet with more healthy fats appeared to be less at risk of developing type 2 diabetes. Learn to eat healthy fats such as monounsaturated and polyunsaturated fats instead of saturated and trans fatty acids and limit your daily fat intake.

PROTEINS

Protein is vital for the growth and maintenance of new cells, organs, and body tissues. It is also important for forming muscles, antibodies, and enzymes. The DASH Diet recommends that you consume about six ounces of meat or alternative protein sources every day to maintain muscle mass. Plant-based protein sources include beans, soybeans, peas, and tofu.

Choose leaner cuts of meat over fatty cuts such as hamburgers and pastrami. Leaner cuts of meat include:

- Boneless, skinless chicken breasts or thighs
- Ground turkey and lean beef
- Poultry such as skinless chicken and turkey breast
- Fish such as salmon, trout, or tuna

Eat no more than one-third of your calories from protein at any given meal, although some experts feel that you should eat more. The DASH Diet is not a low-protein diet, but it urges people to be careful with their dietary intake and avoid foods such as red meat.

SODIUM

The DASH Diet's reduced-sodium prescription is its distinctive feature. The Centers for Disease Control and Prevention (CDC) estimate that Americans ingest 3,400 milligrams of sodium per day, on average.

The recommended daily intake of sodium is 2,300 milligrams (about 5 grams) for people over fifty-one years of age and 1,900 milligrams (about 4.5 grams) for people over seventy years of age.

Choose potassium-rich foods such as low-fat dairy products and vegetables instead of salt at the table. You should not attempt to reduce sodium intake on your own. Consult your doctor or dietitian before reducing your sodium intake. You may consider a medication that can help you lower your blood pressure and lower your risk of heart disease and stroke.

It is important for those following the DASH Diet to note that some food labels can be misleading. Although this diet recommends that you consume less than 3,400 milligrams of sodium per day, food companies can put whatever they want on their nutrition labels.

The DASH Diet plan recommends that you adhere to the limits on sodium consumption and avoid salt substitutes. A number of food companies try to make their products low in sodium by using a chemical called *potassium chloride* instead of sodium chloride. However, this can result in a product with about the same amount of sodium as the original product.

OTHER MINERALS

Eat a variety of vegetables, fruit, and fish rich in essential nutrients. Iron, calcium, fiber, and zinc are other nutrients you should include in your diet. Consume more fish, whole grains, legumes, and nuts. The DASH Diet suggests that you limit your fat intake to no more than 75 grams per day.

A daily intake of 3 ounces of seafood or 3 ounces of meat is adequate. Although it is not clear whether people eat more meat or seafood on the DASH Diet, the average American diet consists mainly of lean red meats and poultry.

Below, you'll find a breakdown of how the DASH Diet compares to other popular diets in their approaches to nutritional content.

	DASH	Mediterranean	Paleo	Keto
Carbs	Emphasis on green leafy vegetables, whole grains, low glycemic index fruits, legumes, and beans	Emphasis on fruits, vegetables, and legumes Emphasis on whole grains	Limited carbohydrates: foods to avoid include grains, potatoes, legumes, and refined sugar	Very limited carbohydrates 5 percent carbohydrates per meal
Fats	Emphasis on fats that improve cholesterol (↑ HDL ↓ LDL) Olive oil, seeds, nuts, fish rich in omega-3 fatty acids Low-fat dairy products	High fat, but an emphasis on healthy fats High monounsaturated to saturated fat ratio	Emphasis on healthy fats from nuts, seeds, and fish rich in omega-3 fatty acids	Emphasis on fats 70–80 percent per meal
Protein	Emphasis on plant proteins like legumes, nuts, and soy products Animal proteins should be limited but can include low-fat dairy, lean meat, eggs, and fish	Relatively limited protein, prefers fish and seafood to other animal proteins	Emphasis on lean meats	20 percent protein per meal Avoidance of excess protein Emphasis on only consuming what is necessary for homeostasis
Sodium	~2300 OR ~1500 mg/day	Avoidance of salt, but no standard limit	Salt avoidance/ limited salt	No salt suggestions

BENEFITS OF THE DASH DIET

Besides reducing hypertension, there are several health advantages that came to light as experts recorded the conditions people experience after choosing to follow this diet. The following are some of the primary benefits of the DASH Diet:

1. **Quick and Easy Liver and Colon Detox:** The DASH Diet originated as a treatment for people with high blood pressure. However, it is now used to treat liver and colon diseases. This is because the diet has been proven to cleanse your liver by eliminating harmful toxins from your body. Sticking to the diet has also helped reduce body weight and improve colon health.

2. **Curb Your Sugar Cravings Without Guilt:** If you have a sweet tooth, the DASH Diet will help you curb your cravings because the diet is low in sugar. Even if you manage to sneak a few unhealthy foods into your diet, you can still lose weight by sticking to the plan. A study published in the *Journal of Nutrition* indicates that healthy salt levels reduce hunger pangs and limit the consumption of sugar-sweetened beverages.

3. **Boost Your Energy Levels:** The DASH Diet is high in potassium and low in sodium, and it provides extra energy. It can be tricky to manage your energy

levels during the early stages of the diet because you may feel tired. That's normal and will get better in time. For now, though, you should drink extra water daily to hydrate your body. This will help you stay energized for longer.

4. **Reach Your Ideal Weight:** If you are overweight and have high blood pressure, the DASH Diet will ensure a healthy body weight. The diet is high in fiber, and research has shown that diets with higher fiber content result in appetite suppression. Therefore, the chances of overeating are slim. Weight loss will also come naturally if you limit your calorie intake. The diet is low in fat and salt, both of which can contribute to weight gain if consumed often or in large amounts.

5. **Fight Inflammation:** Inflammation can lead to cancer and other chronic conditions. A 2011 study published in the *International Journal of Cancer* notes that a high salt intake increases the risk of certain cancers, especially those of the digestive system. While it is not possible to avoid inflammation completely, you can reduce your risk by following the DASH Diet.

6. **Boost Your Heart Health:** The DASH Diet has always been associated with high blood pressure, but recent research has shown that it can also help protect your heart. A study published in the *Journal of the American Medical Association* notes that

individuals who follow the diet tend to have a low risk of heart disease and stroke. This is because the diet lowers blood pressure, which in turn prevents cardiovascular disease, strokes, and heart attacks. Don't forget to consult your doctor before starting a new diet plan.

7. **Easy Blood Sugar Management:** The DASH Diet helps to control your blood sugar levels. This is because it contains a high number of foods with a low glycemic index. This diet forces you to eat fewer bad carbohydrates, improving your overall health. While on the diet, drink plenty of water to keep your blood sugar levels on the right track.

8. **Plan Your Daily Meals on Autopilot:** The DASH nutritional plan is not just another fad diet designed to help you lose weight for a short time. If you stick to the diet, your health will benefit in other ways too. The best part of following the DASH Diet is planning your meals on autopilot as you get used to it. While you can still lead a fulfilling life when following this diet, it may take some time for you to get used to the new meals and healthy eating habits. However, there are other ways that you can make your diet more convenient. For instance, prepare extra portions of healthy food and save them in small containers for easy access. You should also have healthy snacks in your car or bag for easy access when you need a quick energy boost.

9. **Metabolism Booster:** It is proven that the DASH Diet will boost your metabolism. This is because the diet is high in fiber. If you have a sluggish digestive system, the fiber will help to cleanse it and make it function at optimum levels so that your body can burn fat faster. Studies have shown that people who follow the DASH Diet tend to have lower body weights as compared to those who do not follow it.

10. **Improve Your Vitamin K Intake:** Vitamins are essential to the human body. Not all vitamins work the same way, but all of them play important roles. Vitamin K is known to improve health. To meet your needs, you need to consume poultry, beef, fish, and dairy foods. This diet helps you get enough Vitamin K because it emphasizes eating foods that contain high levels of Vitamin K.

3

THE DIET, THE MYTH, THE LEGEND

The DASH Diet works. Results from hundreds of clinical trials have proven the diet's effectiveness. This nutritional plan is a clinically based strategy for lowering blood pressure and reducing your risk of heart disease.

MISCONCEPTIONS SURROUNDING THE DASH DIET

There are many myths or misconceptions about the DASH Diet. To clear up the confusion, here is a list of the most common ones.

Misconception #1: The DASH Diet Is Only for People with High Blood Pressure.

It is a diet plan that can be followed by anyone; the plan will bring benefits to all kinds of people, and everyone is encouraged to follow it. This myth has come about because those who promote the DASH Diet normally advertise it for people who have hypertension or high blood pressure, and take them through a step-by-step process of how to eat according to the diet. As promotional messages for this diet are mainly aimed at people with high blood pressure, some people think that this is just a diet for people who have hypertension or high blood pressure. Whether you have hypertension or not, this is a diet that you should follow.

Misconception #2: "Low-Sodium" and "No-Salt" Are the DASH Diet's Only Focus.

The DASH Diet is a low-sodium diet. Its goal is for people to reduce their sodium intake to a healthy level, which means consuming 2,300 milligrams of sodium or less per day. This myth comes from the misconception that the DASH Diet is only an attempt to lower your sodium intake and nothing else. That isn't true. This nutritional plan focuses on your overall physical health by lowering your blood pressure levels and reducing your risk of illness or disease. This diet does not just focus on lowering your sodium intake; it recommends a healthy diet and lifestyle.

Misconception #3: The DASH Diet Is Unapproachable.

You may feel discouraged to start the DASH Diet if it seems difficult to you. Some people think that following this diet could be boring, and they wouldn't get to eat their favorite foods or snacks. Following the DASH Diet does not mean having to completely change your lifestyle. There are a few small changes that you can make to your current lifestyle and eating habits and still follow the DASH Diet plan. These changes won't drastically affect your everyday life, but they will affect how healthy you are in the long run. That is why it is important to start eating healthier today, even if it is just one small step at a time.

Misconception #4: DASH Is a "Diet" That You Follow Intermittently.

Some people falsely assume that the DASH Diet is equivalent to a fad diet, that you will only be on it for a short period, or that you can break it to eat something else. The DASH Diet is not this kind of short-term diet. This nutritional plan is a way of life that you follow for the long run, even for the rest of your life. You will eat healthier and still keep up with your busy lifestyle. The myth that you have to "go on a diet" and then "break the diet" is not true. When you follow the DASH Diet, you make a lifestyle change for the better. You don't have to follow a strict regimen of restricting your caloric intake or limiting your favorite foods. You can enjoy food while still making sure that it is nutritious and healthy.

FAQS ABOUT THE DASH DIET

Perhaps you have been diagnosed with hypertension and your doctor has recommended the DASH Diet, or maybe you've heard about the diet and want to know more about the plan. Either way, you probably have quite a few questions about this nutritional plan that need answering. I will discuss some of the questions people most often ask about the DASH Diet plan.

Question: How Much Can the DASH Diet Reduce Blood Pressure?

Answer: By limiting sodium intake, the DASH Diet helps to control blood pressure. A high-salt diet raises blood pressure and makes it more difficult for the heart to pump blood. The DASH Diet suggests limiting sodium consumption to 2,300 milligrams per day.

Use a food journal to keep track of how much sodium you eat every day. It is best if you can limit your sodium intake to natural food sources, such as fresh fruit and vegetables. You can find one here at www.nookandnourish.com.

Question: How Effective Is the DASH Diet in Treating Hypertension?

Answer: The DASH Diet was developed in the 1990s. The National Institute of Health began financing various research initiatives in 1992 to determine whether dietary modifications could help with hypertension treatment. To eliminate confounding factors, trial participants were asked to follow the dietary interventions without making any other lifestyle changes. The researchers discovered that dietary changes alone could reduce systolic blood pressure.

Some studies show that this nutritional plan can reduce blood pressure, but others have not shown the efficacy of the diet for hypertension control. The DASH Diet is an overall healthy eating plan which improves chronic disease and lowers health risks. This plan aims to improve your diet by providing suggestions on how to lower sodium intake and reduce fat intake.

Question: Does the DASH Diet Recommend Exercise?

Answer: The DASH Diet recommends getting regular exercise. It is not a DASH Diet plan requirement, only a recommendation. Exercising regularly will help you control your weight and lower blood pressure through increased weight loss and improved heart health.

According to a new study, the DASH Diet combined with aerobic activity resulted in a 30 percent improvement in brain function, as well as decreased blood pressure, improved cardiovascular fitness, and an average weight loss of 19 pounds by the end of the trial. Participants reduced their systolic blood pressure by an average 16 points and their diastolic blood pressure by 10 points on average. When combined with physical activity, the DASH Diet is even more successful at lowering blood pressure. This is not surprising, given the numerous health benefits of exercise. It is recommended that you engage in 30 minutes of moderate activity on most days. Try to find an activity that you enjoy since you are more likely to stick with it.

Question: Is the DASH Diet Safe and Effective?

Answer: Since it was developed in the 1990s, the DASH Diet has been scrutinized by numerous research groups. Researchers have been consistent in their findings that the diet is safe and that it helps people to lower their blood pressure and manage chronic diseases.

For eight running years, the US News & World Report recently voted the DASH Diet, developed by the NIH, the "best overall" diet from around forty reviewed diets. New research reveals that the DASH low-sodium diet controls blood pressure as well as, or better, than several antihypertensive drugs. This nutritional plan was established by researchers supported by the National Heart, Lung, and Blood Institute (NHLBI) of the NIH to prevent and treat high blood pressure, and it has also been shown to reduce blood cholesterol levels.

Question: Why Do Doctors Call It the Best Diet?

Answer: The DASH Diet tied for "best overall" diet this year and was ranked first in the "healthy eating" and "heart disease prevention" categories, with a concentration on vegetables, fruit, whole grains, low-fat dairy, and lean proteins. According to the World Health Organization, hypertension, also known as high blood pressure, is the most common chronic condition worldwide. It is a major risk factor for heart disease, affecting one billion people globally and accounting for one out of every eight fatalities each year. The DASH Diet is an effective and proven way to lower blood pressure and cholesterol, without resorting to medication. Doctors recommend it to their patients as a healthy, natural alternative for treating hypertension.

Question: Is the DASH Diet Safe for Diabetes?

Answer: The DASH Diet plan is an acceptable eating pattern for diabetics. Studies have shown that the diet can improve insulin resistance, hyperlipidemia, and even obesity, in addition to blood pressure regulation. People with diabetes can use the DASH Diet and also take advantage of its potential benefits for hyperlipidemia and blood pressure regulation. Adherence to this nutritional plan can improve insulin sensitivity regardless of weight loss. One study found that when patients with diabetes were put on this diet and lost weight, insulin sensitivity improved by 44 percent when compared to a control group receiving no instruction.

The DASH Diet helps diabetics in numerous ways. It is low in saturated fat, cholesterol, and sodium. It contains a reasonable amount of carbohydrates and recommends healthy sources of fat like olive, canola, peanut, and sunflower oils. This diet provides proper nutrition without increasing your risk of developing diabetes or heart disease.

Working with a doctor is recommended for those with type 2 diabetes mellitus, wanting to try the DASH Diet. It is important to understand that if you do not have diabetes, you can still benefit from following this nutritional plan on a regular basis. Diabetics must follow their doctor's orders on what they should eat or avoid while on the DASH Diet.

Question: What Foods Can You Eat on the DASH Diet?

Answer: The DASH Diet is a lower-sodium diet. That means you can eat healthy foods while still increasing your intake of protein and dietary fiber if you choose to. This nutritional plan is rich in vegetables, fruit, and whole grains. Low-fat or fat-free dairy products, fish, poultry, beans, and nuts are all included.

Foods high in saturated fat, such as fatty meats and full-fat dairy products, are restricted. The diet also prohibits the use of food and beverages heavy in added sugar. Limiting these foods will help you to achieve and maintain a healthy weight.

The DASH Diet recommends eating both plant- and animal-based proteins. Foods such as fish, skinless poultry, beans, eggs, nuts, and seeds factor prominently in the DASH Diet plan as they contain high-quality protein but also have a lower energy density than most other protein sources, making them more satiating. Research indicates that having a higher satiety value is important when considering a sustainable weight loss diet plan.

Question: How Much Sodium Can I Eat in a Day?

Answer: The DASH Diet contains less salt than the typical American diet, which can contain up to 3,400 milligrams of sodium per day. This diet restricts sodium intake to 2,300 milligrams per day. That's about a teaspoon of table salt. The most common sodium sources in the American diet are bread, butter, and cured meats.

The DASH Diet was developed for people with high blood pressure who want to lower their blood pressure without using medication. On the DASH Diet, you can eat practically any food you choose, but it's especially important to eat low-fat dairy and lean meats. Good sources of calcium include dairy products (especially those low in fat), dark green leafy vegetables, tofu, and certain types of fish, such as salmon and canned light tuna in water (check labels for sodium content).

Question: Do I Need Medication with the DASH Diet To Reduce Blood Pressure?

Answer: The DASH Diet does not contain medications to treat high blood pressure. If you are on medications your doctor may recommend that you do not follow the DASH Diet plan until the medications have been discontinued.

There are many effective natural therapies to treat high blood pressure, including some nonpharmaceutical interventions like lifestyle changes and exercise. A diet plan that is low in salt and sugar and rich in nutrients thought to help reduce blood pressure without medication is an appealing alternative to lower the risk of hypertension.

There is no medication to substitute for good nutrition, exercise, and stress reduction. The DASH Diet is a low-sodium plan recognized as one of the most effective ways to treat hypertension since reduced sodium intake can reduce blood pressure without drugs.

Question: Can I Drink Alcohol on the DASH Diet?

Answer: Yes, but studies show that alcohol intake can lead to an increase in blood pressure. The DASH Diet emphasizes a low alcohol intake. Reducing alcohol consumption, according to hypertension treatment guidelines, can lower blood pressure, especially for people who drink more than two drinks per day. In one study published in the *Archives of*

Internal Medicine, one-third of hypertensive patients were also binge drinkers.

Follow the DASH Diet for several weeks before trying to determine whether alcohol adversely affects your blood pressure. A DASH Diet that is lower in sodium and higher in potassium may help offset any adverse effect on blood pressure from alcohol consumption. Alcohol intake should be limited to no more than 1 drink per day for women and two drinks per day for men.

Question: Can I Use the DASH Diet to Lose Weight?

Answer: The DASH Diet is tried and true. If your goal is weight loss, this plan won't melt the pounds off quickly. Still, if you identify the proper calorie level and consistently stick to it, the diet is a safe, effective, and sustainable way to shed pounds and simultaneously improve your health. Weight loss is achieved by creating a calorie deficit. The DASH Diet allows you to eat foods you likely love to eat, so you don't feel deprived, and it's easy to maintain because the foods are rich in nutrients.

The weight loss results from DASH adherence are also associated with the increased physical activity level of 3,500 steps per day versus a sedentary lifestyle (1,600 steps per day), which is related to weight loss in people with metabolic syndrome.

Having a consistent calorie deficit leads to progressive weight loss over time. This is important because reducing weight can bring about significant improvements in health, including better glucose control, reduced risk of cardiovascular disease, cancer prevention, and improved eye health.

While the DASH Diet doesn't result in quick weight loss, it is a healthy eating plan that is based on sound science that may be beneficial to your weight loss goals. The combination of nutrients from fruit and vegetables, along with whole grains and lean proteins, reduces your risk of developing chronic diseases such as diabetes. The reduction in sodium promotes a reduction in blood pressure and cholesterol, which may reduce the risk of stroke and heart attack.

I hope these FAQs helped clarify some of the nitty-gritty details about the DASH Diet. I wrote them to help people get an idea of what they are getting into when they decide to follow the DASH Diet. Most of all, I wrote them in the hope that they will help those who want to learn about the diet and lose weight through exercise and proper nutrition. The DASH Diet can help you achieve your weight loss goals and improve your overall health.

This eating plan is very flexible. You can eat out at restaurants or buy food from any grocery store that has a good selection of fresh vegetables, whole grains, low-fat dairy products, lean meats, and nuts. You can use this plan to lose weight.

The DASH Diet is well-studied and documented, including its ability to reduce blood pressure. If you find that this diet is not running smoothly for you, it may be that you need to tweak it a little bit to make it work better for you, whether that's with the implementation of the plan, or just to help with any problems that may arise during your first several weeks on the diet.

4

28-DAY ACTION PLAN WITH RECIPES

People often jump into a new diet filled with fear and hesitation. With the DASH Diet, there's no reason to be fearful. Most of the diet will sound familiar. It may be prescribed for those with high blood pressure, but it will benefit just about anyone. The diet doesn't stray far from recommendations made in current federal nutrition guidelines. Combining this diet with meal prep allows you even greater control over what you eat and your grocery budget. In this first part, I'll explain the extensive science behind the DASH approach and give you the tools and ingredients you'll need for long-term success.

Planning is a key component of the DASH Diet. Meal prep allows for healthy food choices for every meal and helps you to better manage your grocery budget. Because the diet is based on fresh foods, this shouldn't be an excuse to indulge in processed canned meals. Remember, the whole point of this nutritional plan is to treat yourself well, not create another reason to feel deprived.

To prevent overeating or giving in to temptation, plan your meals in advance and set yourself up for success. Instead of trying to plan your weekly meals on the fly, take an hour or two on Sunday, or the beginning of whatever day works for you, for meal prep. Use shopping lists and preplanned recipes to avoid a frantic run to the grocery store.

A great method is to make a list before going to the store. If you don't plan before going to the grocery store you may buy more food than you need or become distracted by non-healthy foods that aren't right for the DASH Diet. Find healthy and delicious DASH Diet recipes, and write down all the ingredients you need before you go to the store. You won't be tempted by the other food in the grocery store because your mind will be set on the delicious planned meals that comply with the nutritional plan rules.

Eat before going shopping. Similar to the last tip, never shop hungry. When you're hungry, you may develop a wandering eye tempting you to buy more than what's on your list. Also, when you're hungry, you may gravitate toward snacks and processed foods for a quick fix to relieve your hunger. Processed foods are a big nono for the DASH Diet since they're often high in sodium, so avoid temptation by not shopping when you're hungry.

Keep DASH-approved food at home. Diets are all about avoiding temptation. When you keep junk food and sweets next to your healthy options, you're more likely to pick the former. However, if you have the basic food staples recommended by the DASH plan, like grains, vegetables, nuts, and fruits, you're more likely to eat these out of convenience, rather than leave to go to the store and indulge in junk food. Out of sight, out of mind.

Cooking utensils are also an important consideration. Certain tools in the kitchen will be more beneficial to the DASH Diet than others. Here are three kitchen cookware items that you should have in your kitchen: The first is a nonstick pan. This eliminates the need to coat the pan with oil or butter. Since oils and fats are low on the list of food groups you should be eating, it's best to cut down on these fats wherever you can. Next, a steamer. Steamers are great because all they add to your DASH-approved vegetable is water—healthy food cooked to perfection. Lastly, you need a spice mill to grind up whole, natural spices to avoid livening up your meals with salt.

Rinse off canned foods. Canned vegetables are a quick way to buy vegetables, prepare them, and have them last. They're perfectly okay to eat under the DASH Diet. However, the juice in the can carries a lot of excess salt. Get rid of most of this excess by rinsing your vegetables off with water before you eat them.

Don't be afraid to ask questions. It doesn't have to be difficult to eat out and still maintain your diet. If you want to order something off the menu but you're afraid that the salt content may be too high, consult the menu for ingredients. If the menu doesn't list them, you may find deeper nutritional information on the restaurant's website. When in doubt, however, you can always ask the waiter to check with the chef. Many people have dietary restrictions and you won't be considered a burden for asking. This way, you can eat guilt-free and enjoy your meal.

Drink only water. This is a hard feat for some and an easy one for others. If you're a big soda or juice fan, this tip is for you. Sugars, even "fake sugars" like Splenda are put into common prepackaged drinks. You may think buying juice is fine because it's a fruit serving for the day. This may be true, however, there may also be so many added sugars in the drink that the one fruit serving is ultimately canceled out by the sugar in the juice. You can even branch out to sparkling water or tea, but steer clear of drinks with hidden sugars.

Ask for the lunch portion. It's important with the DASH Diet to keep your calories at the expected level. Often restaurants serve large portions and when the food is on your plate, you may feel obligated to eat it. Ask for the lunch portion if you're out to dinner and have them put the rest in a to-go box. Not only are you sticking with your diet this way, but you also are saving money by keeping an extra portion for later.

Fruit for dessert. This tip works both at home and in restaurants. If you're craving something sweet to finish off your meal, turn to dessert. If regular fruit doesn't satisfy you, there are tons of recipes that turn an average dish of fruit into a yummy dessert that still maintains the healthy nutrients provided by the fruit. If at a restaurant, go for a fruit sorbet or parfait. It may have some added sugar, but much less than a devil's food cake would. You'll be sticking to the DASH Diet while enjoying something sweet.

Cut back on meat. This can be a fast or gradual process, depending on how big a meat eater you are. Much of the sodium we try to avoid comes from meat. You don't have to cut out all meat from the start, but gradually reduce your intake. If you eat meat every day, try eating it for six days a week. The same rule can apply to meals, if you eat meat at every meal, take it down to only two meals. For an even more gradual approach, you can just reduce your serving size of meat at each meal.

Meal Prep Works Well with the DASH Diet

Meal prepping may be your secret weapon for putting the DASH Diet into practice. It saves time, reduces waste, and keeps you accountable for your health and wellness goals. Forecasting your menu, getting the ingredients together, and prepping for a full week of meals that you can take on the go eliminates the guesswork of what to eat when you are tired and overwhelmed.

If you're just getting started with meal prepping, you may feel a little anxious. Don't worry, I'm here to guide you. I will show you, step-by-step, how to prepare and streamline your meals so you can stay on track with your DASH Diet plan.

Why Prep?

When you start meal prepping, you may be pleasantly surprised by all the benefits it brings. Meal prepping:

- **Saves time.** Using one day to plan and prepare your meals decreases the time you spend in the kitchen during the rest of the week. That also means less time shopping, cooking, and cleaning, which gives you more time to spend on things you enjoy doing.
- **Reduces waste.** When you plan and prep your meals ahead of time, you can include recipes that feature the same ingredients. This will decrease the amount of food left unused (to possibly spoil) in your refrigerator. Currently, Americans waste one-third of the food they buy each year. Meal prepping could be the start of a sustainable practice for you and the environment.
- **Helps you stick to your diet plan.** Meal prepping allows you to choose foods and flavors that meet your cravings and nutrition goals. Meals that have been frozen can also help you fill the gap when unexpected events occur.

- **Aids in portion control.** Following DASH portion principles and storing your food in individual containers makes it easy to get just what you need and not too much. It also helps you to eat mindfully during your meals—to savor your food rather than devour it out of hunger.
- **Improves your cooking skills.** It goes without saying, but spending time preparing a variety of dishes each week will exponentially increase your confidence in the kitchen.
- **Saves money.** Another benefit of reducing waste, planning, and making fewer last-minute grocery runs is that it saves you money.

Meal Prep Principles

Meal prepping doesn't have to be complicated. The following guidelines can make meal prep easier:

Start Simply

An easy place to start is with readily available ingredients for simple recipes. To ease yourself in, first, focus on prepping a couple of meals a week. Include a few staples and some basics like roast chicken and vegetables, a hearty soup, or a breakfast casserole. As you get more comfortable with the DASH Diet and meal prepping in general, you can expand the number of recipes you prep each week. Later in this book, you'll find additional recipes that will inspire you to add even more variety to your prepared meals.

Use Ingredients Wisely

The beauty of meal prep is that you can use the same ingredients in different ways. When planning, consider not only your main ingredients but also what you use to flavor and add color to your meals. If you use onions and peppers in your morning frittata, plan to include them at lunch in a veggie wrap or a soup. If you used orange juice for a marinade, consider adding oranges to your dinner salad. When choosing fresh herbs, remember that they can enhance the flavor of almost any dish—sauces, marinades, salads, casseroles—don't ever let those herbs go to waste.

Be Flexible and Adaptable

As you start going through the different preps, you'll notice that I encourage variations, substitutions, and additions. I want you to feel comfortable substituting herbs in your seasonings, adding fruit or vegetables to your recipes, and even changing ingredients to some you might prefer or already have on hand. If your recipe calls for apples and you have pears you need to use, feel free to swap them. If you're making a stir-fry, preparing a casserole, roasting vegetables, or baking a frittata, you can always add or substitute leftover vegetables for additional flavor, color, and texture. When it comes to fruit and vegetables in the DASH approach, more is always better.

Be Food Safety Savvy

Understanding the rules of food safety is essential when meal prepping. Although many leftovers may continue to look or smell okay, it is important to know how long you can safely store them. And even though most bacteria that make you ill will not grow in temperatures below 40 degrees F, the bacteria that can cause food to spoil are still active at that temperature. Consider keeping your refrigerator between 35 and 38 degrees F, an ideal temperature to allow an extra day or two of food storage. Freezing meals for later in the week is always a great option.

Caloric Intake Measurements

1600 Calories a Day

- Grains (preferably whole grains or multigrains) = 6 servings
- Vegetables = 3–4 servings
- Fruit = 4 servings
- Nuts, seeds, legumes = 3–4 servings per week
- Fat-free (or low-fat) milk and milk products = 1–2 servings
- Lean meats, fish, and poultry = 3–4 (or fewer) servings
- Fats and oils = 2 servings
- Sweets and added sugars = 3 (or fewer) servings per week

2600 Calories a Day

- Grains (preferably whole grains or multigrains) = 10–11 servings
- Vegetables = 5–6 servings
- Fruit = 5–6 servings
- Fat-free (or low-fat) milk and milk products = 1-2 servings
- Lean meats, fish, and poultry = 6 servings
- Nuts, seeds, legumes = 1 serving
- Fats and oils = 3 servings
- Sweets and added sugars = up to 2 servings a day but not required

3100 Calories a Day

- Grains (preferably whole grains or multigrains) = 12–13 servings
- Vegetables = 6 servings
- Fruit = 6 servings
- Fat-free (or low-fat) milk and milk products = 2–3 servings
- Lean meats, fish, and poultry = 6–9 servings
- Nuts, seeds, legumes = 1 serving
- Fats and oils = 4 servings
- Sweets and added sugars = up to 2 servings a day but not required.

Now, as we get into our recipes, keep in mind that they may contain dairy products. If you're lactose intolerant, you can always replace nonfat milk options with almond or soy milk, cheese with tofu or vegan cheese, and yogurt with coconut yogurt.

BREAKFAST

The first meal of the day is the most important since it kick-starts your metabolism, so make sure to begin each day with a healthy and nutritious meal! This will help you maintain a healthy weight because you won't want to snack as much and your mental focus will improve a lot.

Week One

▷ **Peanut Butter Overnight Oats**

Ready in about: 6 hours 7 minutes
Servings: 1
Nutritional info (per serving): Calories: 453, Protein: 14g, Carbohydrates: 52g, Fat: 21g, Sodium: 228 mg

Ingredients:

Oats:

- ½ cup unsweetened, plain almond milk
- 1 Tbsp. maple syrup

- ½ cup gluten-free rolled oats
- ¾ Tbsp. chia seeds
- 2 Tbsp. natural salted peanut butter

Toppings (Optional):

- Flaxseed meal
- Granola
- Sliced banana
- Strawberries

Instructions:

1. Combine almond milk, chia seeds, peanut butter, and maple syrup (or another sweetener) in a Mason jar or small bowl with a lid. The peanut butter and almond milk do not need to be thoroughly combined.
2. Stir in oats a few more times. Then, using a spoon, press down to ensure that all oats are moistened and submerged in almond milk.
3. Securely cover with a lid or seal and place it in the refrigerator to soak overnight (or for at least 6 hours).
4. Open the following day and serve plain or garnish with desired toppings (see options above).

▷ **Muesli Scones**

Ready in about: 32 minutes
Servings: 8
Nutritional info (per serving): Calories: 299, Protein: 8g,
Carbohydrates: 39g, Fat: 10g, Sodium: 302 mg

Ingredients:

- 2 cups blanched almond flour
- ½ tsp. Celtic sea salt
- ½ tsp. baking soda
- ¼ cup raw sesame seeds
- ¼ cup pistachios, chopped
- 1 large egg
- 2 Tbsp. honey
- ¼ cup dried cranberries
- ¼ cup dried apricots, cut into pieces
- ¼ cup sunflower seeds

Instructions:

1. Combine salt, almond flour, and baking soda in a large mixing bowl.
2. Combine dried fruit, seeds, and nuts in a separate bowl.
3. Combine egg and agave in another small bowl.
4. Combine wet and dry ingredients.

5. Form the dough with your hands.

6. Form dough into a 612 x 612 square that is approximately 3–4 inches thick (16 squares of dough).

7. Bake for 10–12 minutes at 350°F on a baking sheet lined with parchment paper.

8. Serve.

▷ **Healthy Breakfast Cookies**

Ready in about: 30 minutes
Servings: 4–6
Nutritional info (per serving): Calories: 545, Protein: 17.9g, Carbohydrates: 55g, Fat: 31.6g, Sodium: 496 mg

Ingredients:

- 2-¼ cups quick oats
- ½ cup dried cranberries
- ⅔ cup chopped nuts
- 1 cup creamy peanut butter
- ¼ cup honey
- 1 tsp. vanilla extract
- 2 ripe bananas, mashed
- ½ tsp. salt
- 1 tsp. ground cinnamon

Instructions:

1. Preheat the oven to 325°F. Line a baking sheet with parchment paper.
2. In the pot of a stand mixer fitted with a paddle attachment, combine the peanut butter, honey, vanilla extract, mashed bananas, salt, and cinnamon.
3. Combine the oats, dried cranberries, and nuts in a large mixing bowl. Scoop approximately a ¼ cup mounds of cookie dough onto the prepared baking sheet, slightly flattening each cookie. (Because the cookies will not spread during the baking process, they can be packed quite closely together.)
4. Bake for 14–17 minutes, or till golden brown but still soft. Take the cookies out of the oven and cool for 6 minutes on the baking sheet before moving them to a cooling dish to cool completely.

▷ **Slow Cooker Apple Cinnamon Steel-Cut Oatmeal**

Ready in about: 7 hours 12 minutes
Servings: 7
Nutritional info (per serving): Calories: 150, Protein: 5g, Carbohydrates: 4.1g, Fat: 3.5g, Sodium: 178 mg

Ingredients:

- 1 cup uncooked steel-cut oats

- 2 Tbsp. brown sugar
- ½ tsp. cinnamon
- 1 Tbsp. ground flax seed
- 2 apples, peeled, cored, cut into pieces
- 1-½ cups almond milk
- 1-½ cups water
- ¼ tsp. salt
- 1-1/2 Tbsp. butter, cut into 6 pieces (optional)
- Garnishes: chopped nuts, raisins, maple syrup (optional)

Instructions:

1. Coat the interior of a slow cooker measuring 3-1/2 quarts (or larger) with cooking spray. Combine all elements (except the optional toppings) in the slow cooker. Stirring occasionally, cover and cook on low for approximately 7 hours (slow cooker times can vary).
2. Spoon oatmeal into bowls; garnish with desired toppings. Refrigerate leftovers. Freezes extremely well.
3. Reheat single servings as follows: Place 1 cup of cooked oatmeal—substitute ⅓ cup fat-free milk. Stir after 1 minute in the microwave on high. Cook for an additional minute or until hot.

Week Two

▷ Ezekiel Bread French Toast

Ready in about: 22 minutes
Servings: 2
Nutritional info (per serving): Calories: 465, Protein: 13.9g, Carbohydrates: 59.8g, Fat: 18.7g, Sodium: 318 mg

Ingredients:

- ½ cup coconut milk
- 2 Tbsp. coconut sugar
- 1 packet Stevia
- 1 tsp. vanilla
- 4 slices Ezekiel bread
- 2 eggs
- Cinnamon
- A pinch of salt

Instructions:

1. In a huge mixing pot, combine all ingredients except the Ezekiel bread.
2. Each slice of bread should be dipped in the mixture so that the liquid coats both sides.
3. Cook for about 5 minutes per side or until lightly browned.

4. Combine with syrup and serve!

▷ **Open Face Breakfast Sandwich**

Ready in about: 18 minutes
Servings: 4
Nutritional info (per serving): Calories: 349, Protein: 19g,
Carbohydrates: 30.5g, Fat: 17.7g, Sodium: 735 mg

Ingredients:

- 2 cups arugula
- 1 Tbsp. extra-virgin olive oil, divided
- 1-½ tsp. fresh lemon juice
- ½ tsp. salt, divided
- ½ tsp. ground black pepper, divided
- 4 large eggs
- ¾ cup part-skim ricotta cheese
- 4 2-oz. slices whole-wheat country bread
- Cooking spray
- ¼ cup fresh cheese, grated
- 1 tsp. fresh thyme, chopped

Instructions:

1. Coat each side of the bread with cooking spray and toast according to your preference until lightly golden (broil, toaster, or grill).

2. Combination of arugula: Toss the arugula with 2 teaspoons oil, 2 teaspoons juice, ⅛ teaspoon salt, and ¼ teaspoon pepper.

3. Cook the eggs: Heat 1 teaspoon of olive oil in a nonstick saute pan over medium heat. Cook for 2 minutes after cracking the eggs into the pan. Cover and continue cooking for another 2 minutes or until the whites are set. Take the pan off the heat. Add ¼ teaspoon of salt, ricotta, fresh grated cheese, and thyme.

4. Assemble the sandwich as follows: Add a layer of the ricotta mixture and arugula salad to the toast, followed by a cooked egg. Season with salt and pepper to taste.

5. Serve right away.

▷ **Mushroom Spinach Omelet**

Ready in about: 26 minutes
Servings: 1
Nutritional info (per serving): Calories: 427, Protein: 28.3g, Carbohydrates: 12g, Fat: 29g, Sodium: 265 mg

Ingredients:

- 1 Tbsp. olive oil
- 1-½ cup fresh spinach
- 5 baby Bella mushrooms, sliced

- Cooking spray
- 1 whole egg
- 2 egg whites
- ¼ cup red onion, sliced
- 1 oz. goat cheese
- Green onions, diced (optional garnish)

Instructions:

1. Preheat a medium skillet over moderately high heat. To the pan, add olive oil and red onions. Cook, occasionally stirring, for 2–4 minutes, or until the onions are translucent.
2. Sauté the sliced mushrooms in the pan until they begin to brown slightly, around 4–5 minutes.
3. Add spinach to the pan. Saute for 3 minutes, or till the spinach is wilted. Season with sea salt and freshly ground pepper. Place aside.
4. Preheat a small skillet over medium heat. Coat with nonstick cooking spray.
5. Put one whole egg and two egg whites into a small bowl. Whisk to combine.
6. In a small pan, add the egg mixture. Allow one minute for the mixture to set. Gently work your way around the pan edges with a spatula. Then lift the skillet and gently tilt it down and around in a circular motion to let the "runny" eggs in the center

cook along the newly cleaned edges. Continue in this manner for another minute.

7. To one side of the omelet, add the mushroom and spinach mixture and top with crumbled goat cheese. Gently fold the other side of the omelet over the mushroom and spinach side using your spatula. Allow to settle for 30 seconds before gently transferring the omelet to a plate. Serve garnished with green onions.

Week Three

▷ **Healthy Egg Bake**

Ready in about: 42 minutes
Servings: 6
Nutritional info (per serving): Calories: 200, Protein: 16.7g, Carbohydrates: 3.3g, Fat: 13.6g, Sodium: 637 mg

Ingredients:

- ¼ cup almond milk
- 1 tsp. Dijon mustard
- 10 oz. frozen spinach, chopped
- 12 large eggs, beaten
- ¼ tsp. ground black pepper
- ¼ tsp. ground nutmeg
- ½ cup shredded sharp cheddar cheese (optional)

- 1 tsp. dried thyme
- 1 tsp. kosher salt

Instructions:

1. Preheat the oven to 350°F. Using an oil spray, coat a 9-inch pie pan or cast-iron skillet.
2. Squeeze spinach to remove excess moisture and place in the prepared pie pan.
3. Mix the eggs and milk in a bowl. Whisk in mustard, thyme, salt, pepper, and nutmeg. Pour the egg mixture over the spinach. Garnish with cheddar.
4. Move to the oven and bake for approximately 30 minutes, or until the mixture is set in the center. Remove from the oven and allow to cool for 5–10 minutes. Serve in six wedges.

▷ **Smoked Salmon Avocado Toast**

Ready in about: 8 minutes
Servings: 2
Nutritional info (per serving): Calories: 308, Protein: 25g, Carbohydrates: 7g, Fat: 20.4g, Sodium: 856 mg

Ingredients:

- 3 oz. smoked salmon
- 1 pinch salt-free garlic & herb seasoning

- 2 slices whole grain bread
- ½ of an avocado

Instructions:

1. Toast 2 slices of bread and spread the avocado evenly between the two.
2. Season the avocado and top with wild salmon.

▷ **Make-Ahead Vegetarian Breakfast Salad with Eggs**

Ready in about: 23 minutes
Servings: 1
Nutritional info (per serving): Calories: 258, Protein: 8g, Carbohydrates: 20g, Fat: 21.9g, Sodium: 261 mg

Ingredients:

- 1-½ cups baby arugula
- ⅛ tsp. sea salt
- 2 large free-range eggs
- ⅛ tsp. black pepper
- 1 Tbsp. lemon juice
- 1-½ tsp. olive oil
- ½ cup avocado
- ¾ cup grape tomatoes
- ¼ cup red onion

Instructions:

1. In a serving pot, whisk together the lemon juice and oil. Top with avocado, tomatoes, onion, and arugula in that order. *IMPORTANT: Do not toss to combine.* Refrigerate overnight.
2. Toss the salad together in the morning and season with salt.
3. Heat an organic cooking spray in a large (PFOA-free) nonstick skillet over medium heat. Cook until the eggs are sunny-side-up or to the desired doneness, about 4 to 5 minutes.
4. Set the eggs on the salad. (Or, if desired, garnish the salad with sliced hard-boiled eggs.) Season with freshly ground black pepper.

▷ **Instant Pot Steel-Cut Oats**

Ready in about: 15 minutes
Servings: 6
Nutritional info (per serving): Calories: 130, Protein: 4.5g, Carbohydrates: 23.2g, Fat: 2.2g, Sodium: 10 mg

Ingredients:

- 2-½ cups steel-cut oats
- 2 cinnamon sticks
- 7 cups water

Instructions:

1. In an Instant Pot, combine steel-cut oats, water, and cinnamon sticks.
2. Secure the Instant Pot's lid and vent. Cook in the Instant Pot for 6 minutes on the manual setting.
3. Allow 20 minutes for the pressure to naturally release after the Instant Pot beeps.
4. Remove the lid, discard the cinnamon sticks, and stir the oats to absorb any remaining liquid.
5. Assemble with the toppings of your choice. (A combination of blueberries, sliced almonds, and honey is delicious.)

Week Four

▷ **Banana Muffins**

Ready in about: 41 minutes
Servings: 6
Nutritional info (per serving): Calories: 303, Protein: 6g, Carbohydrates: 45.3g, Fat: 11.8g, Sodium: 112 mg

Ingredients:

- ¼ cup canola oil
- ½ tsp. pure vanilla extract
- ½ cup all-purpose flour

- 2 overripe bananas
- ½ cup whole-wheat flour
- 1 tsp. baking powder
- ¼ tsp. salt
- ½ tsp. ground cinnamon
- ¼ cup granulated sugar
- 1 egg
- 2 Tbsp. chocolate chips (optional)

Instructions:

1. Preheat the oven to 350°F. Coat a six-muffin tin with nonstick cooking spray.
2. Place bananas in a medium mixing bowl. Mash and stir them with a fork until completely mashed.
3. Combine the sugar and bananas in a large mixing bowl. Then, add the egg and combine.
4. Stir the oil and vanilla extract into the banana mixture.
5. In a medium bowl, combine the flours. Combine the salt, baking powder, and cinnamon in another medium bowl. Whisk dry ingredients together, then add it to the banana mixture. Gently stir until the dry ingredients are just combined.
6. Distribute batter evenly among six muffin cups. Chocolate chips can be sprinkled on top if desired.
7. Bake for 20–23 minutes, or until the muffins are lightly browned.

8. Enjoy!

▷ Ham & Egg Breakfast Burrito

Ready in about: 12 minutes
Servings: 1
Nutritional info (per serving): Calories: 158, Protein: 19g, Carbohydrates: 22g, Fat: 4.1g, Sodium: 683 mg

Ingredients:

- 2 dashes bottled hot sauce
- 2 Tbsp. mild salsa
- ¼ cup frozen egg product
- 1 (8 in.) high-fiber whole-wheat tortilla, warmed
- 1 oz. low-fat, reduced-sodium cooked ham, sliced

Instructions:

1. Coat a small, unheated, nonstick skillet lightly with cooking spray. Heat salsa, ham, and hot sauce over medium-high heat for 3 minutes. Reduce the heat to medium-low and add the egg product. Cook, occasionally stirring, until the mixture begins to set on the bottom and around the sides. Lift and gather the partially cooked egg mixture with a spatula or large spoon, allowing the uncooked portion to flow underneath. Cook for an extra 3–5 minutes, or

until the egg mixture is set but still glossy and moist.

2. Distribute the egg mixture evenly across the tortilla.
3. Roll up the tortilla.

▷ **Overnight Oatmeal**

Ready in about: 16 minutes
Servings: 1
Nutritional info (per serving): Calories: 346, Protein: 11g, Carbohydrates: 53g, Fat: 12g, Sodium: 53 mg

Ingredients:

- ½ cup assorted fresh fruit
- 2 Tbsp. chopped walnuts, toasted
- 3 Tbsp. fat-free milk
- ⅓ cup old-fashioned oats
- 3 Tbsp. reduced-fat plain yogurt
- 1 Tbsp. honey

Instructions:

1. Combine oats, milk, yogurt, and honey in a small container or Mason jar. Fruit and nuts can be added as garnishes.
2. Refrigerate for at least 24 hours before serving.

LUNCH

Calculate the nutrition info on the back of the food packaging. Aim for foods with less than 5 percent of your daily value sodium allowance. High-sodium foods are those that contain at least 20 percent of the recommended daily intake of sodium. Always remember to double-check the sodium content and other nutrition information based on the serving size.

Week One

▷ **Tomato-Garlic Lentil Bowls**

Ready in about: 35 minutes
Servings: 6
Nutritional info (per serving): Calories: 295, Protein: 22g, Carbohydrates: 48g, Fat: 3g, Sodium: 419 mg

Ingredients:

- 1 Tbsp. olive oil
- 3 cups water
- ¼ cup lemon juice
- 3 Tbsp. tomato paste
- ¾ cup fat-free, plain Greek yogurt
- 2 onions, chopped
- 4 garlic cloves, minced

- 2 cups dried brown lentils, rinsed
- 1 tsp. salt
- ½ tsp. ground ginger
- ½ tsp. paprika
- ¼ tsp. pepper
- Chopped tomatoes and minced fresh cilantro (optional)

Instructions:

1. In a large saucepan over medium heat, sauté onions in oil for 2 minutes. Stir in lentils, seasonings, and water and bring to a boil. Decrease to low heat and cook, covered, for 25–30 minutes, or until lentils are tender.
2. Add lemon juice and tomato paste and bring to a boil. Serve with yogurt, tomatoes, and cilantro, if desired.

▷ **California Sushi Rolls**

Ready in about: 1 hour 16 minutes
Servings: 8 rolls
Nutritional info (per serving): Calories: 36, Protein: 2g, Carbohydrates: 6.7g, Fat: 1g, Sodium: 30 mg

Ingredients:

- 2 cups sushi rice, rinsed and drained
- 8 nori sheets
- 1 cucumber, seeded and julienned
- 3 oz. imitation crab meat sticks, julienned
- 1 ripe avocado, peeled and julienned
- 2 cups water
- ¼ cup rice vinegar
- 2 Tbsp. sugar
- ½ tsp. salt
- 2 Tbsp. sesame seeds, toasted
- 2 Tbsp. black sesame seeds
- Reduced-sodium soy sauce (optional)

Instructions:

1. Combine rice and water in a large saucepan. Bring to a boil over high heat. Reduce to low heat, cover, and cook for 15–20 minutes, or until the water is absorbed and the rice is tender. Take the pan off the heat. Allow to stand for 10 minutes, covered.
2. Meanwhile, mix the sugar, vinegar, and salt in a small bowl until the sugar dissolves.
3. In a large shallow bowl, transfer rice; drizzle with vinegar mixture. Stir the rice in a slicing motion with a wooden paddle or spoon to cool slightly. Keep moist by covering with a damp cloth. (You may

prepare the rice mixture up to 2 hours ahead and store it at room temperature, covered with a damp towel. Do not refrigerate.)

4. On a plate, sprinkle toasted and black sesame seeds; set aside. Arrange a sushi mat on a work surface in such a way that it rolls away from you; wrap in plastic wrap. Arrange ¾ cup rice on a piece of plastic. Press rice into an 8-inch square using moistened fingers and place a nori sheet on top.

5. Arrange a small amount of cucumber, crab, and avocado on the nori sheet, about 1-1/2 in. from the bottom edge. Roll the rice mixture over the filling, lifting and compressing the mixture with the bamboo mat as you roll. Remove the plastic wrap as you roll.

6. Remove the mat and roll the sushi over the sesame seed-covered plate. Wrap in plastic wrap. Continue with the remainder of the ingredients to make 8 rolls. Each should be cut into eight pieces. If desired, garnish with soy sauce, wasabi, and sliced ginger.

▷ **Strawberry Blue Cheese Steak Salad**

Ready in about: 36 minutes
Servings: 4
Nutritional info (per serving): Calories: 290, Protein: 30g, Carbohydrates: 12g, Fat: 14g, Sodium: 452 mg

Ingredients:

- 1 lb. beef top sirloin steak
- ½ tsp. salt
- ¼ tsp. pepper
- 2 tsp. olive oil
- 2 Tbsp. lime juice
- ¼ cup crumbled blue cheese
- ¼ cup chopped walnuts, toasted
- Reduced-fat balsamic vinaigrette
- 10 cups romaine lettuce, torn
- 2 cups fresh strawberries, halved
- ¼ cup red onion, sliced

Instructions:

1. Season each side of the steak with salt and pepper. Heat the oil over medium heat in a large pan. Cook for 5–7 minutes on each side or until it reaches the desired degree of doneness(for medium-rare, a thermometer should read 135°; for medium, 140°; and for medium-well, 145°). Remove from the pan and set aside to cool for 5 minutes. Prepare the steak by cutting it into bite-size strips and tossing it with lime juice.
2. Combine romaine lettuce, strawberries, and onion on a platter and top with the steak. Cheese and

walnuts should be sprinkled on top. Accompany with vinaigrette.

▷ Turkey and Vegetable Barley Soup

Ready in about: 41 minutes
Servings: 6
Nutritional info (per serving): Calories: 209, Protein: 22g, Carbohydrates: 23g, Fat: 4g, Sodium: 662 mg

Ingredients:

- 6 cups reduced-sodium chicken broth
- 2 cups cooked turkey breast, cubed
- 2 cups fresh baby spinach
- ½ tsp. pepper
- 1 Tbsp. canola oil
- 5 carrots, chopped
- 1 onion, chopped
- ⅔ cup quick-cooking barley

Instructions:

1. In a large saucepan, heat the oil over medium-high heat. Add carrots and onion; cook, stirring until the carrots are crisp-tender, 4–5 minutes.
2. Stir in the barley and the broth and bring it to a boil. Reduce heat and simmer covered, until the carrots

and barley are tender, 10–15 minutes. Stir in the
turkey, spinach, and pepper; heat through.

Week Two

▷ **Corn, Rice, and Bean Burritos**

Ready in about: 38 minutes
Servings: 8
Nutritional info (per serving): Calories: 327, Protein: 14.2g,
Carbohydrates: 52g, Fat: 7g, Sodium: 500 mg

Ingredients:

- 1 Tbsp. canola oil
- 1-½ cups cooked brown rice
- 8 flour tortillas (8 in.), warmed
- ¾ cup shredded reduced-fat cheddar cheese
- ½ cup reduced-fat plain yogurt
- 2 green onions, sliced
- ½ cup salsa
- 1-⅓ cups fresh corn
- 1 onion, chopped
- 1 medium green pepper, sliced
- 2 garlic cloves, minced
- 1-½ tsp. chili powder
- ½ tsp. ground cumin
- 15 oz. black beans, rinsed and drained

Instructions:

1. Heat the oil over medium-high heat in a huge pan. Add corn, onion, and pepper; cook and stir until tender. Add garlic, chili powder, and cumin and cook for 1 minute longer. Add the beans and rice; heat through.
2. Spoon ½ cup of filling across the center of each tortilla. Top with cheese, yogurt, and green onions. Turn the bottom and sides of the tortilla over the filling and roll up. Serve with salsa.

▷ **Easy Southwestern Veggie Wraps**

Ready in about: 36 minutes
Servings: 6
Nutritional info (per serving): Calories: 297, Protein: 12g, Carbohydrates: 53g, Fat: 3g, Sodium: 525 mg

Ingredients:

- 1 cup cooked brown rice, cooled
- ⅓ cup fat-free sour cream (optional)
- ½ tsp. ground cumin
- ½ tsp. chili powder
- 15 oz. black beans, rinsed and drained
- 2 large tomatoes, seeded and diced
- 1 cup frozen corn, thawed

- ½ tsp. salt
- 6 romaine leaves
- 6 whole-wheat tortillas (8 in.)
- ¼ cup fresh cilantro, minced
- 2 shallots, chopped
- 1 jalapeño pepper, seeded and chopped
- 2 Tbsp. lime juice

Instructions:

1. Place all the ingredients except the romaine and tortillas in a large bowl; toss to combine.
2. To serve, place the romaine on the tortillas, top with the bean mixture, and roll up, securing them with toothpicks if desired. Cut in half.

▷ **Shrimp & Nectarine Salad**

Ready in about: 36 minutes
Servings: 4
Nutritional info (per serving): Calories: 253, Protein: 24g, Carbohydrates: 27g, Fat: 7g, Sodium: 448 mg

Ingredients:

- 1-½ tsp. Dijon mustard
- 1-½ tsp. honey
- 1 Tbsp. fresh tarragon, minced

- ⅓ cup orange juice
- 3 Tbsp. cider vinegar
- 4 tsp. canola oil, divided
- 8 cups mixed salad greens, torn
- 2 nectarines, cut into 1-inch pieces
- 1 cup grape tomatoes, halved
- ½ cup red onion, chopped
- 1 cup fresh or frozen corn
- 1 lb. uncooked shrimp, peeled and deveined
- ½ tsp. lemon-pepper seasoning
- ¼ tsp. salt

Instructions:

1. Whisk orange juice, vinegar, mustard, and honey together in a small bowl until smooth. Combine with the tarragon.
2. Heat 1 tsp. of oil in a large pan over medium-high heat. Cook and stir for 1–3 minutes, or until the corn is crisp-tender. Take it out of the pan.
3. Season the shrimp with lemon pepper and salt to taste. Heat the remaining oil in the same skillet over medium-high heat. Add shrimp and cook, occasionally stirring, for 3–4 minutes, or until the shrimp turns pink. Combine with the corn.
4. Combine the remaining ingredients in a large mixing bowl. Drizzle ⅓ cup dressing over the salad and toss to coat. Distribute the mixture evenly between four

plates and drizzle the remaining sauce over the shrimp mixture. Serve right away.

Week Three

▷ **Thai Chicken Pasta Skillet**

Ready in about: 35 minutes
Servings: 6
Nutritional info (per serving): Calories: 404, Protein: 26g, Carbohydrates: 43g, Fat: 14g, Sodium: 432 mg

Ingredients:

- 2 cups cooked chicken, shredded
- 1 cup Thai peanut sauce
- 1 cucumber, halved, seeded, and sliced
- 6 oz. uncooked whole-wheat spaghetti
- 2 tsp. canola oil
- 10 oz. sugar snap peas, trimmed
- 2 cups carrots, julienned
- Fresh cilantro, chopped (optional)

Instructions:

1. Cook the spaghetti according to package directions; drain.
2. Meanwhile, in a large skillet, heat the oil over medium-high heat. Add snap peas and carrots; stir-fry for 6–8 minutes or until crisp-tender. Add the chicken, peanut sauce, and spaghetti. Heat through and toss to combine.
3. Transfer to a serving plate and top with cucumber and cilantro, if desired.

▷ **Italian Sausage-Stuffed Zucchini**

Ready in about: 58 minutes
Servings: 6
Nutritional info (per serving): Calories: 207, Protein: 18g, Carbohydrates: 17g, Fat: 8g, Sodium: 485 mg

Ingredients:

- 6 medium zucchini
- ⅓ cup fresh parsley, minced
- 2 Tbsp. fresh oregano, minced
- 2 Tbsp. fresh basil, minced
- ¼ tsp. pepper
- ¾ cup shredded part-skim mozzarella cheese
- 1 lb. Italian turkey sausage links, casings removed

- 2 medium tomatoes, seeded and chopped
- 1 cup panko bread crumbs
- ⅓ cup grated Parmesan cheese
- Fresh parsley, minced (optional)

Instructions:

1. Preheat the oven to 350°F. Cut each zucchini in half lengthwise. Scoop the pulp out, leaving a ¼-inch border. Chop up the pulp. In a large microwave-safe dish, arrange zucchini shells. Microwave covered, in batches on high for 2–3 minutes or until crisp-tender.
2. Cook the sausage and zucchini pulp in a large skillet over medium heat for 6–8 minutes, or until the sausage is no longer pink, crumbling the link; drain. Combine the sausage with the tomatoes, bread crumbs, Parmesan cheese, herbs, and pepper in a large mixing bowl. Fill zucchini shells halfway with the mixture.
3. Place in two 13 x 9-inch ungreased baking pans. Wrap and bake for 15–21 minutes or until the zucchini is tender. Sprinkle mozzarella cheese on top. Bake, wrapped, for an additional 5–8 minutes, or until the cheese is melted. Sprinkle with additional minced parsley, if desired.

▷ **Mimi's Lentil Medley**

Ready in about: 45 minutes

Servings: 8

Nutritional info (per serving): Calories: 226, Protein: 11g, Carbohydrates: 29g, Fat: 7g, Sodium: 404 mg

Ingredients:

- 1 cup dried lentils, rinsed
- 3 Tbsp. olive oil
- 2 tsp. honey
- 1 tsp. dried basil
- 1 tsp. dried oregano
- 4 cups fresh baby spinach, chopped
- 4 oz. crumbled feta cheese (optional)
- 2 cups water
- 2 cups fresh mushrooms, sliced
- 1 medium cucumber, cubed
- 1 medium zucchini, cubed
- 1 small red onion, chopped
- ½ cup soft sun-dried tomato halves, chopped
- ½ cup rice vinegar
- ¼ cup fresh mint, minced
- 4 bacon strips, cooked and crumbled (optional)

Instructions:

1. In a small saucepan, combine lentils and water. Bring to a boil. Decrease to low heat and cook covered, for 20–25 minutes, or until the lentils are tender. Drain and rinse them thoroughly with cold water.
2. Transfer the mixture to a large bowl. Combine the mushrooms, cucumber, zucchini, onion, and tomatoes in a medium bowl. Whisk together vinegar, mint, oil, honey, basil, and oregano in another small bowl.
3. Drizzle over the lentil blend and toss to coat with the dressing. Toss in spinach, cheese, and bacon, if desired.

▷ Tomato Green Bean Soup

Ready in about: 55 minutes
Servings: 9
Nutritional info (per serving): Calories: 59, Protein: 5g, Carbohydrates: 10g, Fat: 1g, Sodium: 535 mg

Ingredients:

- 1 cup onion, chopped
- 3 cups fresh tomatoes, diced
- ¼ cup fresh basil, minced
- ½ tsp. salt

- ¼ tsp. pepper
- 1 cup carrots, chopped
- 2 tsp. butter
- 6 cups reduced-sodium chicken
- 1 lb. green beans, cut into pieces
- 1 garlic clove, minced

Instructions:

1. Sauté the onion and carrots in butter for 6 minutes in a large saucepan. Bring to a boil, stirring in the broth, beans, and garlic. Decrease to low heat and cover; cook for 20 minutes, or until the vegetables are tender.
2. Combine the tomatoes, basil, salt, and pepper in a medium bowl. Cover and continue simmering for an additional 5 minutes.

Week Four

▷ **Cannellini Bean Hummus**

Ready in about: 12 minutes
Servings: 10
Nutritional info (per serving): Calories: 79, Protein: 4g, Carbohydrates: 8g, Fat: 3g, Sodium: 114 mg

Ingredients:

- 2 garlic cloves, peeled
- 15 oz. can cannellini beans, rinsed and drained
- ¼ cup tahini
- 3 Tbsp. lemon juice
- 1-½ tsp. ground cumin
- ¼ tsp. salt
- ¼ tsp. crushed red pepper flakes
- 2 Tbsp. fresh parsley, minced
- Pita bread, cut into wedges
- Assorted fresh vegetables

Instructions:

1. Place the garlic into a food processor; cover and process until minced. Cover and process the beans, tahini, lemon juice, cumin, salt, and pepper flakes until smooth.
2. Move the mixture to a small bowl and season with salt and pepper. Stir in the parsley. Refrigerate until you're ready to serve it with pita wedges and a variety of fresh vegetables.

▷ **Shrimp Orzo with Feta**

Ready in about: 33 minutes

Servings: 4

Nutritional info (per serving): Calories: 407, Protein: 34g,
Carbohydrates: 40g, Fat: 11g, Sodium: 307 mg

Ingredients:

- 1-¼ lb. uncooked shrimp, peeled and deveined
- 2 Tbsp. fresh cilantro, minced
- ¼ tsp. pepper
- ½ cup crumbled feta cheese
- 1-¼ cups uncooked whole-wheat orzo pasta
- 2 Tbsp. olive oil
- 2 garlic cloves, minced
- 2 tomatoes, chopped
- 2 Tbsp. lemon juice

Instructions:

1. Cook the orzo following package instructions.
   Meanwhile, in a large skillet, heat the oil over
   medium heat. Add the garlic and cook, stirring, for 1
   minute. Add tomatoes and lemon juice and bring to a
   boil. Stir in the shrimp and reduce the heat; simmer
   uncovered, until the shrimp turns pink, 4–5 minutes.

2. Drain the orzo. Add the orzo, cilantro, and pepper to the shrimp mixture; heat through. Sprinkle with feta cheese.

▷ **California Quinoa**

Ready in about: 36 minutes
Servings: 4
Nutritional info (per serving): Calories: 311, Protein: 12g, Carbohydrates: 42g, Fat: 10g, Sodium: 353 mg

Ingredients:

- 1 Tbsp. olive oil
- 1 medium tomato, chopped
- ½ cup crumbled feta cheese (optional)
- ¼ cup Greek olives, finely chopped
- 2 Tbsp. fresh basil, minced
- ¼ tsp. pepper
- 1 cup quinoa, rinsed and drained well
- 2 garlic cloves, minced
- 1 zucchini, chopped
- 2 cups water
- ¾ cup canned garbanzo beans, rinsed and drained

Instructions:

1. Heat the oil in a large pan over medium-high heat. Add the quinoa. Cook and stir for 2–3 minutes, or until the quinoa is lightly browned.
2. Bring to a boil, stirring in the zucchini and water. Reduce the heat to low and cook covered, for 12–15 minutes, or until the liquid is absorbed. Add the remaining ingredients and heat until they are thoroughly combined.

DINNER

According to a national sleep survey, most people are in bed by eleven at night. With this in mind, it is strongly advised that you finish eating by eight o'clock, which allows for digestion before sleep and helps prevent calorie-dense night-time grazing.

There are so many delicious DASH Diet dinner recipes to choose from. So here are a few of my top picks and some simple ways to jazz up your vegetables.

Week One

▷ **Roasted Chicken Thighs with Peppers & Potatoes**

Ready in about: 58 minutes

Servings: 8

Nutritional info (per serving): Calories: 309, Protein: 25g, Carbohydrates: 25g, Fat: 11g, Sodium: 221 mg

Ingredients:

- 2 lb. red potatoes
- 3 tsp. fresh rosemary, minced
- 8 boneless chicken thighs
- ½ tsp. salt
- ¼ tsp. pepper
- 2 large sweet red peppers
- 2 large green peppers
- 2 medium onions
- 2 Tbsp. olive oil, divided
- 4 tsp. fresh thyme, minced and divided

Instructions:

1. Preheat the oven to 450°F. Potatoes, peppers, and onions should all be cut into 1-inch pieces. In a roasting pan, arrange vegetables. Drizzle 1 tablespoon of oil over the vegetables and sprinkle

with 2 teaspoons of thyme and 2 teaspoons of rosemary, tossing to coat. Place the chicken on top of the vegetables. Brush the remaining oil onto the chicken and sprinkle it with the remaining thyme and rosemary. Season the chicken and vegetables with salt and pepper.

2. Roast for 35–42 minutes, or until a thermometer inserted in the chicken registers 170°F, and the vegetables are tender.

▷ **Peppered Tuna Kabobs**

Ready in about: 36 minutes
Servings: 4
Nutritional info (per serving): Calories: 206, Protein: 30g, Carbohydrates: 20g, Fat: 2g, Sodium: 50 mg

Ingredients:

- 2 Tbsp. parsley, coarsely chopped
- 2 Tbsp. lime juice
- ½ cup frozen corn, thawed
- 4 green onions, chopped
- 1 jalapeño pepper, seeded and chopped
- 2 sweet red peppers, cut into pieces
- 1 mango, peeled and cut into 1-inch cubes
- 1 lb. tuna steaks, cut into 1-inch cubes
- 1 tsp. coarsely ground pepper

Instructions:

1. To make the salsa, combine the first five ingredients in a small bowl; set aside.
2. Pepper the tuna. Alternately thread red peppers, tuna, and mango onto four metal or soaked wooden skewers.
3. Place skewers on a greased grill rack. Cook, covered, over medium heat, turning occasionally, for 10–12 minutes, or until the tuna is slightly pink in the center (medium-rare) and the peppers are tender. Serve alongside the salsa.

▷ **Apple-Cherry Pork Medallions**

Ready in about: 37 minutes
Servings: 4
Nutritional info (per serving): Calories: 408, Protein: 32g, Carbohydrates: 46.8g, Fat: 10g, Sodium 470 mg

Ingredients:

- 1 lb. pork tenderloin
- 1 Tbsp. olive oil
- 1 large apple, sliced
- ⅔ cup unsweetened apple juice
- 3 Tbsp. dried tart cherries
- 1 Tbsp. honey

- 1 Tbsp. cider vinegar
- 8-1/2 oz. ready-to-serve brown rice
- 1 tsp. fresh rosemary, minced
- 1 tsp. fresh thyme, chopped
- ½ tsp. celery salt

Instructions:

1. In a large nonstick skillet, heat the oil over medium-high heat. Cut the tenderloin crosswise into 12 slices and sprinkle with rosemary, thyme, and celery salt. Brown both sides of the pork then remove them from the pan.
2. Combine apple, apple juice, cherries, honey, and vinegar in the same skillet. Bring to a boil, constantly stirring to dislodge browned bits from the bottom of the pan. Decrease the heat to low and cook, wrapped, for 3–4 minutes, or until the apple is tender.
3. Return the pork to the pan, turning to coat with the sauce; cook for 3–4 minutes longer covered, or until the pork is tender. Meanwhile, prepare the rice as directed on the package. Serve with the pork mixture.

▷ **Asparagus Turkey Stir-Fry**

Ready in about: 26 minutes

Servings: 4

Nutritional info (per serving): Calories: 206, Protein: 29g, Carbohydrates: 5g, Fat: 8g, Sodium: 204 mg

Ingredients:

- 2 Tbsp. canola oil, divided
- 1 lb. fresh asparagus, trimmed
- 2 oz. sliced pimientos, drained
- 2 tsp. cornstarch
- ¼ cup chicken broth
- 1 Tbsp. lemon juice
- 1 tsp. soy sauce
- 1 lb. turkey breast tenderloins, cut into strips
- 1 garlic clove, minced

Instructions:

1. Mix the broth, lemon juice, cornstarch, and soy sauce in a small bowl until smooth, then set aside. Stir-fry turkey and garlic in 1 Tbsp. of oil in a large skillet or wok till the meat is no longer pink. Then, remove from the heat and keep it warm.
2. In the remaining oil, stir-fry the asparagus and pimientos until crisp-tender. Stir the broth mixture

into the pan and cook it for 1 minute, or until it has slightly thickened. Add the turkey back into the pan and heat through.

Week Two

▷ **Sweet Onion & Sausage Spaghetti**

Ready in about: 37 minutes
Servings: 4
Nutritional info (per serving): Calories: 335, Protein: 18g, Carbohydrates: 41g, Fat: 11g, Sodium: 378 mg

Ingredients:

- 2 tsp. olive oil
- 1 sweet onion, sliced
- 1 pint cherry tomatoes, halved
- ½ cup basil leaves, thinly sliced
- 6 oz. uncooked whole-wheat spaghetti
- ¾ lb. Italian turkey sausage links, casings removed
- ½ cup half-and-half cream
- Shaved Parmesan cheese (optional)

Instructions:

1. Cook the spaghetti according to the package instructions. Meanwhile, in a huge nonstick skillet

over medium heat, cook the sausage in the oil for 5
minutes. Add the onion and cook for an extra 8–10
minutes until the meat has lost its pink color and the
onion is tender.
2. Add the tomatoes and basil and heat through. Then
add the half and half cream and bring to a boil. Drain
the spaghetti and toss with the sausage mixture.
Garnish with cheese if desired.

▷ **Chicken & Goat Cheese Skillet**

Ready in about: 32 minutes
Servings: 2
Nutritional info (per serving): Calories: 252, Protein: 31g,
Carbohydrates: 8g, Fat: 10g, Sodium: 447 mg

Ingredients:

- ½ lb. boneless chicken breasts, cut into pieces
- 1 cup fresh asparagus, sliced
- 1 garlic clove, minced
- 3 plum tomatoes, chopped
- 3 Tbsp. milk
- 2 Tbsp. Herbed fresh goat cheese, crumbled
- ¼ tsp. salt
- ⅛ tsp. pepper
- 2 tsp. olive oil
- Cooked rice or pasta, heated

- Goat cheese (optional)

Instructions:

1. Toss the chicken with salt and pepper to taste. Sauté the chicken in oil over medium-high heat until it is no longer pink, 4–6 minutes. Remove the chicken from the pan and set it aside to keep warm.
2. Cook and stir the asparagus in a skillet for 1 minute over medium-high heat. Add the garlic and cook, constantly stirring, for 30 seconds. Add the tomatoes, milk, and 2 tablespoons cheese; cook covered, over medium heat for 2–3 minutes, or until the cheese begins to melt.
3. Combine with the chicken and serve alongside rice or pasta. Additional cheese, if desired, may be sprinkled on the top.

▷ **Bow Ties with Sausage & Asparagus**

Ready in about: 37 minutes
Servings: 6
Nutritional info (per serving): Calories: 248, Protein: 18g, Carbohydrates: 28g, Fat: 6g, Sodium: 441 mg

Ingredients:

- 9-1/2 oz. Italian turkey sausage links
- 1 onion, chopped
- 3 garlic cloves, minced
- ¼ cup shredded Parmesan cheese
- 8 oz. uncooked whole-wheat bow tie pasta
- 1 lb. fresh asparagus, trimmed and cut into pieces
- Shredded Parmesan cheese (optional)

Instructions:

1. Cook the pasta in a 6-quart stockpot following the package instructions, adding asparagus during the final 2–3 minutes of cooking. Return the pasta and asparagus to the pot, reserving ½ cup of the pasta water.
2. Meanwhile, cook the sausage, onion, and garlic in a large skillet over medium heat until the sausage is no longer pink, 6–9 minutes, breaking the sausage into huge crumbles. Combine it in a stockpot. Stir in a ¼ cup cheese and reserved pasta water. If desired, top with additional cheese.

Week Three

▷ Cod and Asparagus Bake

Ready in about: 37 minutes
Servings: 4
*Nutritional info (per serving): Calories: 142, Protein: 24g,
Carbohydrates: 6g, Fat: 3g, Sodium: 125 mg*

Ingredients:

- 4 cod fillets
- 1 lb. fresh thin asparagus, trimmed
- 1 Tbsp. lemon juice
- 1½ tsp. grated lemon zest
- ¼ cup grated Romano cheese
- 1 pint cherry tomatoes, halved

Instructions:

1. Preheat the oven to 375°F. Place the cod and
   asparagus in a 15 x 10 x 1-in. baking pan brushed
   with oil. Add the tomatoes, and cut sides down.
   Brush the fish with lemon juice and sprinkle it with
   lemon zest. Sprinkle the fish and vegetables with
   Romano cheese. Bake until the fish just begins to
   flake, about 12 minutes.

2. Remove the pan from the oven; preheat the broiler.
    Broil the cod mixture 3–4 in. from the heat until the
    vegetables are lightly browned, 2–3 minutes.

▷ **Weeknight Chicken Chop Suey**

Ready in about: 38 minutes
Servings: 6
*Nutritional info (per serving): Calories: 303, Protein: 26g,
Carbohydrates: 34g, Fat: 6g, Sodium: 237 mg*

Ingredients:

- 4 tsp. olive oil
- 1 cup unsweetened pineapple tidbits, drained
- 8 oz. sliced water chestnuts, drained
- 1 medium tart apple, chopped
- 1 lb. boneless chicken breasts
- ½ tsp. dried tarragon
- ½ tsp. dried basil
- 1 cup cold water, divided
- 1 Tbsp. unsweetened pineapple juice
- ½ tsp. dried marjoram
- ½ tsp. grated lemon zest
- 1-½ cups carrots, chopped
- ½ cup onion, chopped
- 1 tsp. reduced-sodium teriyaki sauce
- 2 Tbsp. cornstarch

- 3 cups cooked brown rice

Instructions:

1. Heat the oil in a huge cast-iron or other heavy skillet over medium heat. Cook the chicken, herbs, and lemon zest, until lightly browned.
2. Combine the five ingredients and bring to a boil, stirring in a ¾ cup of water, pineapple juice, and teriyaki sauce. Reduce to low heat and cover; cook for 10–15 minutes, or until the chicken is no longer rosy and the carrots are tender.
3. Combine the cornstarch and the remaining water in a mixing bowl. Gradually incorporate the flour into the chicken mixture.
4. Bring to a boil; cook and stir for approximately 2 minutes, or until thickened. Serve alongside the rice.

▷ **Stir-Fry Rice Bowl**

Ready in about: 34 minutes
Servings: 4
Nutritional info (per serving): Calories: 306, Protein: 13g, Carbohydrates: 40g, Fat: 10g, Sodium: 364 mg

Ingredients:

- 1 Tbsp. canola oil

- 2 medium carrots, julienned
- 1 Tbsp. chili garlic sauce
- 4 large eggs
- 4 cups cooked brown rice
- 1 tsp. sesame oil
- 1 medium zucchini, julienned
- ½ cup baby portobello mushrooms, sliced
- 1 cup bean sprouts
- 1 cup fresh baby spinach
- 1 Tbsp. water
- 1 Tbsp. reduced-sodium soy sauce

Instructions:

1. Heat the canola oil in a large pan over medium-high heat. Cook the carrots, stirring, for 3–5 minutes, or until they are crisp-tender. Add the bean sprouts, spinach, water, soy sauce, and chili sauce and cook, stirring, until the vegetables are wilted. Remove from the heat; keep warm.
2. In a large skillet with high sides, add 2–3 inches of water. Bring to a boil, then reduce to a gentle simmer. Break the eggs into a small bowl one at a time. Holding the bowl close to the water's surface, softly slip the egg into the water.
3. Cook, uncovered, for 3–5 minutes, or until the whites are completely set, and the yolks begin to thicken but remain soft. Use a slotted spoon to

remove the eggs.

4. Serve over rice and drizzle with sesame oil. Top each serving with a poached egg.

▷ **Green Curry Salmon with Green Beans**

Ready in about: 37 minutes

Servings: 4

Nutritional info (per serving): Calories: 367, Protein: 25g, Carbohydrates: 29g, Fat: 16g, Sodium: 340 mg

Ingredients:

- 4 salmon fillets
- 1 cup light coconut milk
- 1 Tbsp. green curry paste
- ¾ lb. fresh green beans, trimmed
- 1 tsp. sesame oil
- 1 tsp. sesame seeds, toasted
- Lime wedges
- 1 cup uncooked instant brown rice
- 1 cup reduced-sodium chicken broth
- ⅛ tsp. pepper

Instructions:

1. Preheat the oven to 400°F. Place the salmon into an 8-inch square baking dish. Combine the coconut

milk and curry paste in a small bowl and pour over the salmon. Bake, wrapped, for 15–20 minutes, or until the fish begins to flake easily with a fork.

2. Meanwhile, combine the rice, broth, and pepper in a small saucepan and bring to a boil. Decrease to low heat and cover for 5 minutes. Take off the heat and set aside for 6 minutes.

3. Put a steamer basket over 1 inch of water in a large saucepan. Place green beans in the basket and bring the water to a boil. Reduce to low heat and steam, covered, for 7–10 minutes, or until the beans are crisp-tender. Combine the sesame oil and sesame seeds in a bowl.

4. Serve the salmon with rice, beans, and lime wedges. Pour the coconut sauce evenly over the salmon.

Week Four

▷ **Chicken with Celery Root Puree**

Ready in about: 53 minutes
Servings: 4
Nutritional info (per serving): Calories: 329, Protein: 38g, Carbohydrates: 28g, Fat: 7g, Sodium: 348 mg

Ingredients:

- 1 onion, chopped

- 2 garlic cloves, minced
- 4 boneless chicken breast halves
- 3 cups butternut squash, peeled and chopped
- ⅔ cup unsweetened apple juice
- ½ tsp. pepper
- ¼ tsp. salt
- 3 tsp. canola oil, divided
- 3 cups celery root, peeled and chopped

Instructions:

1. Sprinkle the chicken with salt and pepper. In a large nonstick skillet, heat 2 teaspoons of oil over medium heat. Brown chicken on both sides, then remove from the pan.
2. In the same pan, heat the remaining oil over medium-high heat. Add the celery root, squash, and onion. Cook, stirring until the squash is crisp-tender. Add garlic and cook for 1 minute longer.
3. Return the chicken to the pan and add the apple juice. Bring to a boil. Reduce the heat and simmer covered, for 12–15 minutes or until a thermometer inserted in the chicken reads 165°F.
4. Remove the chicken; keep warm. Allow the vegetable mixture to cool slightly before processing it in a food processor until smooth. Return the mixture to the pan and heat through. Serve with the chicken.

▷ **Pepper Ricotta Primavera**

Ready in about: 28 minutes
Servings: 6
*Nutritional info (per serving): Calories: 230, Protein: 12g,
Carbohydrates: 31g, Fat: 6g, Sodium: 88 mg*

Ingredients:

- 1 cup part-skim ricotta cheese
- ½ cup fat-free milk
- 4 tsp. olive oil
- 1 medium zucchini, sliced
- 1 cup frozen peas, thawed
- ¼ tsp. dried oregano
- ¼ tsp. dried basil
- 6 oz. fettuccine, cooked and drained
- 1 garlic clove, minced
- ½ tsp. crushed red pepper flakes
- 1 green pepper, julienned
- 1 sweet red pepper, julienned
- 1 sweet yellow pepper, julienned

Instructions:

1. Whisk together ricotta cheese and milk, then set
   aside. In a large skillet, heat the oil over medium

heat. Sauté the red pepper flakes and garlic for 1 minute.

2. Combine the next seven ingredients. Cook and stir over medium heat for about 5 minutes, or until the vegetables are crisp-tender.

3. Combine the cheese mixture and fettuccine; garnish with vegetables. Toss to coat. Serve right away.

▷ **Beef and Black Bean Spaghetti Squash**

Ready in about: 37 minutes
Servings: 4
Nutritional info (per serving): Calories: 402, Protein: 27g, Carbohydrates: 51g, Fat: 11g, Sodium: 314 mg

Ingredients:

- 1 medium spaghetti squash
- ¾ lb. lean ground beef
- 4 small garlic cloves, minced
- 15 oz. no-salt-added black beans, rinsed and drained
- 2 cups fresh kale, chopped
- ¼ cup plain Greek yogurt
- ½ cup red onion, chopped
- 2 Tbsp. yellow mustard
- 3 tsp. Louisiana-style hot sauce

Instructions:

1. Trim the squash ends and cut in half lengthwise. Seeds should be discarded. Place the squash, cut side down, on a trivet insert, in a 6 qt. electric pressure cooker.
2. Fill the pressure cooker with 1 cup of water and lock the lid. Adjust to high and pressure cook for 7 minutes. Rapidly release pressure, then set the squash aside.
3. In a large skillet over medium heat, crumble beef and cook with onion until it is no longer pink, 4–6 minutes; drain. Cook 1 minute longer. Add mustard, hot sauce, beans, kale, and garlic. Cook, occasionally stirring until the kale is wilted, about 2–3 minutes.
4. Separate spaghetti squash strands with a fork, then combine with meat mixture. Dollop servings with Greek yogurt.

SNACKS

Fruit and other low-fat foods provide an abundance of flavor and variety. Fruit in its natural state requires little or no preparation. Dried fruit is an excellent option for carrying around or keeping in your car.

Week One

▷ Double Chocolate Peanut Butter Cookies

Ready in about: 47 minutes

Servings: 24

Nutritional info (per serving): Calories: 237, Protein: 6.3g, Carbohydrates: 31.7g, Fat: 10g, Sodium: 146 mg

Ingredients:

- 1 cup creamy peanut butter
- 1-½ cups all-purpose flour
- ¼ cup cocoa powder
- 1 tsp. baking soda
- ¼ tsp. salt
- 1 cup semi-sweet chocolate chips
- ½ cup butter, softened
- ½ cup granulated sugar
- ½ cup packed brown sugar
- 2 eggs
- 1 Tbsp. vanilla extract

Instructions:

1. Preheat the oven to 350°F. Line two baking pans with parchment paper.

2. In a large mixing pot, add the peanut butter, butter, sugar, and brown sugar. Beat together until smooth and creamy (best if using a stand mixer or hand mixer).

3. Add the eggs and vanilla extract and continue to mix until the ingredients are well combined.

4. In a small mixing bowl, whisk the flour, cocoa powder, baking soda, and salt. Stir the flour mixture into the butter and sugar mixture and mix until they are well combined. Then stir in the chocolate chips.

5. Use a cookie dough scooper or use your hands to mold the dough into 1-inch balls. Roll in white granulated sugar, if desired, and place on a baking sheet.

6. Use a fork to press down on each dough ball to slightly flatten it and create a criss-cross pattern.

7. Bake for 8–9 minutes. Allow to cool on the baking sheet for a few minutes and then transfer to a wire rack.

8. These keep well in an airtight holder for a couple of days.

▷ **Cheesy Cauliflower Breadsticks**

Ready in about: 55 minutes
Servings: 12
Nutritional info (per serving): Calories: 67, Protein: 6.3g, Carbohydrates: 4g, Fat: 3g, Sodium: 340 mg

Ingredients:

- 1 large egg
- ¼ cup fresh basil, chopped
- ¼ cup fresh parsley, chopped
- 1 garlic clove, minced
- 1 tsp. salt
- ½ tsp. pepper
- 1 head of cauliflower, cut into florets
- ½ cup shredded cheese
- ½ cup grated Parmesan cheese
- ½ cup shredded cheddar cheese
- Marinara sauce (optional)

Instructions:

1. Preheat the oven to 425°F. Process cauliflower in a food processor in batches until finely ground. Then, microwave in a microwave-safe pot covered, on high for about 8 minutes, or until tender.
2. Wrap cauliflower in a clean kitchen towel and squeeze dry when cool enough to handle. Return to the bowl.
3. Combine the cheeses in a separate bowl. Stir half of the cheese mixture into the cauliflower, reserving the remainder.
4. Combine the first six ingredients in a small bowl, then stir into the bowl with the cauliflower.

5. Shape the cauliflower mixture into an 11 x 9-inch rectangle on a parchment-lined baking sheet. Bake for 21–25 minutes, or until the edges are golden brown.

6. Top with the reserved cheese and bake for 10–12 minutes, or until melted and bubbly. Serve with marinara sauce, if desired.

Week Two

▷ **Chia Seed Protein Bites**

Ready in about: 20 minutes
Servings: 10
Nutritional info (per serving): Calories: 73, Protein: 3.9g, Carbohydrates: 9g, Fat: 3g, Sodium: 14mg

Ingredients:

- 1-½ cups quick-cooking oats
- ½ cup honey
- ¼ cup vanilla protein powder
- ½ cup almond butter
- ½ cup chia seeds
- ¼ cup unsweetened, shredded coconut

Instructions:

1. In a huge bowl, combine the first six ingredients. Refrigerate for an hour, or until the mixture is firm enough to roll.
2. Shape into 1-½-inch balls. Roll in coconut if desired. Store in the refrigerator.

▷ **Yogurt & Honey Fruit Cups**

Ready in about: 18 minutes
Servings: 6
Nutritional info (per serving): Calories: 98, Protein: 3g, Carbohydrates: 23g, Fat: 0g, Sodium: 22 mg

Ingredients:

- ½ cups cut-up fresh fruit
- ½ tsp. grated orange zest
- ¼ tsp. almond extract
- ¾ cup vanilla yogurt
- 1 Tbsp. honey

Instructions:

1. Divide the fruit among six individual serving bowls.
2. Combine the yogurt, honey, orange zest, and almond extract; spoon over the fruit.

Week Three

▷ **Garden Vegetable Cornbread**

Ready in about: 45 minutes
Servings: 9
Nutritional info (per serving): Calories: 151, Protein: 6g, Carbohydrates: 28g, Fat: 2g, Sodium: 567 mg

Ingredients:

- ¾ cup whole-wheat flour
- 2-½ tsp. baking powder
- 1 cup yellow cornmeal
- 1 tsp. fresh chives, minced
- ¾ tsp. salt
- ¾ cup carrots, shredded
- ¼ cup sweet red pepper, chopped
- ¼ cup poblano pepper, seeded and chopped
- 2 large eggs
- 1 cup milk
- 1 Tbsp. honey

Instructions:

1. Preheat the oven to 400°F. Whisk together the first five ingredients. In a separate bowl, whisk together the eggs, milk, and honey until smooth. Stir into the

cornmeal mixture until just moistened. Then, fold in the carrots and peppers.

2. Transfer to an 8-inch square, greased, baking pan. Bake for 22–26 minutes, or until a toothpick inserted in the center comes out clean. Serve immediately.

▷ **Healthy Avocado Pineapple Muffins**

Ready in about: 52 minutes
Servings: 12
Nutritional info (per serving): Calories: 209, Protein: 6g, Carbohydrates: 26g, Fat: 9g, Sodium: 190 mg

Ingredients:

- 2 Tbsp. canola oil
- ½ tsp. baking powder
- ½ tsp. baking soda
- ⅔ cup ripe avocado, cubed
- 3 large eggs
- ¼ cup honey
- ½ tsp. ground cinnamon
- ¾ cup chopped pecans, toasted and divided
- 8 oz. unsweetened crushed pineapple, undrained
- 2 cups all-purpose flour
- ½ tsp. salt

Instructions:

1. Preheat the oven to 375°F. Beat the avocado in a large mixing bowl until only small lumps remain. Combine the eggs, honey, and oil in a mixing bowl and beat until smooth, then combine with the pineapple. Separately, whisk together the flour, salt, baking powder, baking soda, and cinnamon. Stir into the avocado mixture until just moistened, then incorporate ½ cup of pecans.

2. Fill 12 greased or foil-lined muffin cups halfway with the batter and sprinkle the remaining ¼ cup of pecans on top. Bake for 22–26 minutes, or till a toothpick put in the center comes out clean. Allow 5 minutes for cooling before transferring to a wire rack. Serve immediately.

Week Four

▷ **Chunky Banana Cream Freeze**

Ready in about: 23 minutes
Servings: 3
Nutritional info (per serving): Calories: 182, Protein: 4g, Carbohydrates: 29g, Fat: 6g, Sodium: 35 mg

Ingredients:

- 5 bananas, peeled and frozen
- 3 Tbsp. raisins
- ⅓ cup almond milk
- 1 tsp. vanilla extract
- ¼ cup chopped walnuts
- 2 Tbsp. unsweetened shredded coconut
- 2 Tbsp. creamy peanut butter

Instructions:

1. In a food processor, add the milk, coconut, bananas, peanut butter, and vanilla; cover and process until smooth.
2. Transfer to a freezer container and add walnuts and raisins; stir to combine. Prior to serving, place in the freezer for 2–4 hours.

▷ **Hummus & Veggie Wrap**

Ready in about: 16 minutes
Servings: 1
Nutritional info (per serving): Calories: 236, Protein: 8g, Carbohydrates: 33g, Fat: 7g, Sodium: 415 mg

Ingredients:

- 2 Tbsp. hummus
- 1 whole-wheat tortilla (8 in.)
- 2 Tbsp. alfalfa sprouts
- 2 Tbsp. carrot, shredded
- 1 Tbsp. balsamic vinaigrette
- ¼ cup mixed salad greens, torn
- 2 Tbsp. sweet onion, chopped
- 2 Tbsp. cucumber, thinly sliced

Instructions:

1. Spread the hummus onto the tortilla.
2. Layer with salad greens, onion, cucumber, sprouts, and carrots.
3. Drizzle with vinaigrette.
4. Roll up tightly.

5

GROCERY GUIDE

The National Institute of Health promotes the DASH Diet, which is a well-balanced lifelong approach to healthy eating, based on nutrient-rich whole foods. This next portion of the book will teach you how to achieve and maintain a healthy weight while also decreasing your blood pressure and cholesterol levels using this nutritional plan. Hypertension, also known as high blood pressure, affects about one billion people globally. High blood pressure not only raises the risk of stroke and heart disease, but it is also the main cause of death. The DASH Diet aims to minimize salt in your diet while increasing calcium, magnesium, potassium, and fiber intake through a wide variety of whole foods that lower blood pressure. This diet is a healthy eating plan, which includes vegetables, fruit, whole grains, fish, lean meats, low-fat dairy, and healthy fats. The American Heart Association recommends this diet, which has been scientifically proven to decrease blood pressure and cholesterol. The DASH Diet is also a popular weight-reduction diet as research shows that it is highly effective in aiding weight loss.

If you want to use the DASH Diet, the type of food you buy is the most important factor. Finding the perfect foods for your diet might be tough, but I've put together a list of suggestions to assist you. Make a list of the essential foods you'll need for your meals before you go grocery shopping. As you make your shopping list, keep the following suggestions in mind:

1. Plan your meals around seasonal fruit and vegetables to save time and effort in the search for out-of-season produce.
2. Choose whole-grain foods like whole wheat bread, whole wheat pasta, brown rice, quinoa, and barley.
3. For delicious and filling protein and fiber, include beans, peas, or lentils.
4. Include skinless poultry, seafood, lean meats, and tofu.
5. Include fat-free or low-fat dairy products (soy milk, almond milk, or Lactaid milk if you're lactose intolerant).
6. Choose low-sodium canned vegetables, tomato sauce, beans, broth, and soup.
7. Try low-sodium dressings and condiments.

8. Buy fresh whenever possible and read the nutrition facts label to compare calories.

9. Be prepared to make a lifestyle change. The DASH Diet is not a quick fix, this is a diet plan that you must continue over your lifetime.

10. To reach three servings of dairy products, try adding a low-fat dairy product at each meal.

11. When choosing your vegetables, use fresh or low-sodium (no salt added) canned or frozen vegetables. Don't use table salt or butter when serving these vegetables.

12. Read food labels thoroughly and choose low-sodium and low-fat (especially those low in saturated fat) foods.

13. If you feel the need for something sweet, snack on dried fruit.

14. Use substitutes for some food items. For example, use whole wheat pasta or brown rice instead of standard noodles and white rice. For desserts, opt for fruit or other healthy foods instead of sweets and high-calorie items.

15. Exercise is always an essential part of any healthy lifestyle. Eating healthy foods like those of the DASH Diet plan is only part of the diet.

16. Try using a food journal to help you keep track of what you eat.

This grocery guide is meant to help you plan what healthy foods you should consume on the DASH Diet. You have the freedom to mix and match foods from each category for that given week so that you don't have to eat the same thing every day. If you are going to stick to the DASH Diet for life, you should aim to eat a wide variety of foods.

DASH Diet Food List

As a newbie on the diet, you probably want to explore various alternatives to foods with which you are unfamiliar. Below is a comprehensive list of foods and ingredients you can use safely with the DASH Diet in the next 28 days.

Disclaimer: Please be aware of food allergens (such as shellfish and peanuts) included in this food list.

FRUITS AND VEGETABLES

- Apples
- Artichokes
- Arugula
- Asparagus
- Avocados
- Bananas
- Bell peppers
- Berries
- Broccoli

- Brussels sprouts
- Cabbage
- Carrots
- Cauliflower
- Celery
- Collard greens
- Corn
- Cucumbers
- Eggplant
- Grapes
- Green Beans
- Kale
- Lemons
- Lettuce
- Limes
- Mushrooms
- Onions
- Pears
- Pineapple
- Potatoes
- Radishes
- Raisins
- Snow peas
- Spinach
- Sprouts
- Squash
- Swiss chard

MEAT AND SEAFOOD

- Chicken
- Eggs
- Fish
- Salmon
- Shrimp
- Turkey

BREAD AND GRAINS

- Barley
- Brown Rice
- Oats
- Whole grain cereal
- Whole wheat bread
- Whole wheat pasta
- Whole wheat tortillas
- Wild rice

NUTS AND SEEDS

- Almonds
- Cashews
- Peanuts
- Pecans
- Pumpkin seeds

- Walnuts

DAIRY

- Cottage cheese
- Fat-free milk
- Reduced-fat cheeses
- Sour cream

FOR LACTOSE INTOLERANT

- Almond milk
- Cashew cheese
- Coconut yogurt
- Extra virgin olive oil
- Hemp milk
- Oat milk
- Soy milk

6

WEIGHT LOSS WITH THE DASH DIET

Although it was developed to lower blood pressure, this diet plan brings several other health benefits. The DASH Diet is recommended for weight loss because it is low in calories, rich in water and fiber, and low in saturated fats. An important caveat to emphasize is that when you put the DASH Diet into practice, you must include a balanced amount of protein-rich foods to keep your muscle mass at an optimal level and avoid metabolic slowdown. Many of the foods included in this diet contain plenty of antioxidants and powerful sources of fats that are healthy for your heart, reducing oxidation and inflammation. A diet rich in vegetables and fruit also supports healthy intestinal flora for good health. The DASH Diet plan is a complete lifestyle program that improves heart health by lowering blood pressure and cholesterol while at the same time promoting weight loss and overall healthy eating.

Lose Weight with the DASH Diet

Recent research has shown that it is possible to lose weight if you follow the DASH Diet and reduce your overall sodium consumption. In a study of 810 people, one-third of them learned to reduce sodium consumption and to follow the DASH Diet daily, at the minimum calorie level, without forgetting healthy physical activity. Within 18 months, the participants had lost weight.

I'd also like to remind you that the DASH Diet likely contains more fruit, vegetables, and whole grains than the diet you're used to. Because this diet is heavy in fiber, it may induce bloating and diarrhea in some people. To avoid these issues, gradually increase your consumption of fruit, veggies, and whole grains.

If you're concerned about reducing your sodium intake, worry not: the secret to reducing the amount of salt in your diet is to eat intelligently. Only a small amount of the salt we consume is represented by cooking salt, meaning the salt contained in a salt shaker, and there are only small amounts of sodium in non-preserved foods. It follows that the main source of sodium is processed and preserved foods, so it is really important to read the labels carefully and choose products with low-sodium content.

While embarking on a healthy diet will take you on a journey to excellent health and well-being, other factors contribute to a healthy mind and body. The real key to safe and successful weight loss is to adopt a lifestyle that will suit your individual needs and that you can maintain for life. If you want to lose weight, the first step is exercise. One important part of exercise is lifting weights. If you're new to fitness, don't start lifting weights right away because it can exhaust your muscles. Begin by speed walking, which is a great and simple approach to burning calories. Walking for just thirty minutes a day can help with weight loss. Add strength training to your program once you've become acclimated to practicing cardio.

Adding weight lifting to your gym routine can help you build more muscle and aid with fat loss. Weight lifting also helps to strengthen your bones, heart, and other vital organs essential for your overall health. You can burn more calories by completing squats to lift your body weight with just your legs. Your metabolism can also stay raised in the twenty-four hours after you have finished your resistance training session. This, likewise, assists in weight loss.

With that being said, your diet will make or break your weight loss. The goal is to reduce calories, but eating only salad and chicken won't help you reach your goals. Opt for lean protein sources with each meal, fruit or veggies throughout the day, and whole grains instead of refined carbs; these are easy ways to make healthier choices while still losing weight and feeling great.

Another lifestyle change that you could adopt is to ditch added sugars. This harmful substance can make you feel sluggish and cause cravings for more unhealthy snacks. Sugary drinks are major contributors to unhealthy weight gain and health problems like diabetes and heart disease, so the best choice is to swap your soda for water. Foods like candy, soda, and baked goods contain lots of added sugars which are very low in nutrients and high in calories.

It is essential to remain hydrated throughout the day. Water is a vital nutrient that aids in the maintenance of good health by maintaining the right balance of water and nutrients in the body. Drinking enough water can help you to lose weight by filling you up on less food, in addition to being pure and additive-free. According to a study published in the *New England Journal of Medicine*, those who drink water before meals consume fewer calories throughout the day. The right amount of water allows you to feel full even when you've eaten less food, and it's also more satisfying since you're less likely to overeat or choose foods that aren't good for your diet. According to one study of nearly 9,500 adults, those who were not well hydrated had higher BMIs and many were overweight.

Studies have also shown that eating more fiber-rich foods helps with weight loss. The more fiber you eat, the fewer calories you'll absorb with each meal, resulting in weight loss. Fiber is a type of carbohydrate that the body partially digests before absorbing, so it has a lower glycemic index than other carbohydrate types. Since fiber slows down digestion and absorption without affecting satiety levels, you will feel fuller faster and for longer.

Healthy fats are an essential part of a diet, and they also aid in weight loss. In fact, some studies show that substituting dietary fats for lean protein can help you to lose more weight. It's important to choose the right types of healthy fats since some fats are high in calories and unhealthy substances. Studies show that eating healthy fats can make you feel fuller, leading to reduced snacking between meals. Moderate amounts of healthy fat such as natural monounsaturated and polyunsaturated fatty acids (found in olive oil, fish oil, and nuts) also help to lower cholesterol in the blood, reducing your risk of developing heart disease. Nutrition experts commonly recommend limiting fat to 30 percent of your daily caloric intake.

Ideal sources of healthy fats are low in saturated and trans fats and contain omega-3 fatty acids. An ounce of olive oil contains about 13 grams of fat, which is about the amount found in two eggs. Reducing the amount of saturated fats will help you lose weight, but it's important to limit the amount of trans fats as well. These are harmful fats that are commonly found in processed foods and restaurants, causing increased levels of LDL (low-density lipoprotein) cholesterol.

Please don't deprive yourself of your favorite foods entirely. Instead, eat them in moderation by cutting out unnecessary portions. Eating everything in moderation means you won't feel deprived and will allow you to continue enjoying your favorite foods.

Sleep is essential for your overall health, and research has shown that the right amount of sleep plays an important role in healthy weight loss. Sleep deprivation can affect your judgment and decision-making, which can result in unhealthy choices when it comes to food. Getting an adequate amount of sleep helps you to improve your diet by reducing cravings for unhealthy foods and compulsive eating between meals. Sleep is also responsible for the production of hormones that regulate appetite, making your body less responsive to food cues. However, one study of 817 people found no association between getting the recommended amount of sleep and weight loss. One study showed that children who slept fewer than eight hours a day ate 15 percent more calories than those who got eight to nine hours. Getting sufficient sleep can also help improve your metabolism, which translates to more calories burned throughout the day.

Volunteer work or other activities that keep you busy and active are great ways to lose weight. Research shows that people who are already involved in physical activity tend to eat healthier and manage their weight better. Exercising is also an effective way to reduce stress, helping you to feel happier and reducing the urge to overindulge in unhealthy foods.

4 CORE COMPONENTS TO WEIGHT LOSS ON THE DASH DIET

1. Protein Intake

Foods rich in protein that comply with DASH Diet guidelines include poultry, fish, beans, and lentils. You will also benefit from eating food like low-fat cheese and skim milk in moderation and choosing whole grains in place of refined grains. You only need to consume one to two cups of low-fat cottage cheese or soy products each day to meet your protein requirements.

2. Intake of Healthy Fats

This component is actually the same as the Mediterranean diet. The key here is to eat healthy fats, which are essential for health and help with weight loss. Instead of eating refined, processed oils like margarine, you can use healthier varieties of fat at the grocery store. These could include olive oil, nuts, seeds, avocado, and coconut oil. Consuming healthy fats is important because they promote weight loss while providing essential nutrients.

3. Mineral Intake

Focus on eating plenty of whole grains, fruit, and vegetables to cover your mineral requirements. People on this diet tend to eat a lot of whole grains because they are rich in magnesium, calcium, and fiber. Make sure you choose a variety of greens as they are good sources of calcium.

4. Low Carbohydrate Intake

Choose foods that are low in carbohydrates and limit your intake of sugars. This will help you lose weight and keep it off. Check food labels to determine which foods contain large amounts of carbohydrates. It is most important to choose complex carbohydrates over simple carbohydrates whenever possible.

PORTION DISTORTION

No matter how healthily you're eating, you can still put on weight if you're eating too much. Nowadays food portion sizes are far bigger than they were 25–30 years ago, which means most people consume more calories than they realize. In fact, many of us no longer know what makes a normal portion. This is a problem known as portion distortion. Regain some portion control with these simple tips:

- Eat off smaller plates and bowls. You will have a smaller portion and still feel satisfied.
- Aim for two portions of vegetables. This will cover your plate with low-calorie ingredients, leaving less room for higher-calorie foods.
- Avoid eating fast. It takes about 20–25 minutes for your stomach to tell your brain it is full. When you eat fast, it is easier to overeat.
- Avoid eating in front of the TV, as you could eat more without noticing or enjoying your food.

PORTION MANAGEMENT

SYMBOL	MEASUREMENT	FOODS	CALORIES
	THUMB 2 Tbsp	Peanut Butter (Dairy) Cheese	170 100
	HANDFUL 1 oz	Nuts Dried Fruit	170 85
	PALM 3 oz	Meat	160
	FIST 1 cup	Rice Fruit Veggies	200 75 40

What to Do if You Can't Lose Weight

If you're finding it difficult to lose weight with a healthy approach like the DASH Diet, you'll need to develop some strategies. Here are a few suggestions:

- Eat smaller portions.
- Increase your fiber consumption.
- Exercise for at least thirty minutes a day to maintain weight, or sixty minutes a day to lose weight.

DASH Diet and Physical Exercise

By combining the DASH Diet with regular physical activity programs such as running and swimming, you can lose weight and maintain long-term results. Thirty minutes a day of moderate-intensity physical activity may be a true solution. If your blood pressure is slightly higher than normal, you may just walk at an active pace for about thirty minutes every day, without having to rely on medication. Even if you don't suffer from high blood pressure, physical activity can help you stay healthy. If you sit for long periods, even if you have normal blood pressure, you are more likely to suffer from high blood pressure, weight gain, obesity, and diabetes later on.

If you suffer from chronic health problems, or your family has a history of developing heart disease at a young age, you must seek advice from your doctor before starting an exercise program.

To start a physical activity program, walk around the block for 15 minutes once in the morning and once in the evening. Build your program little by little and set new goals, so you don't lose your motivation. Keep in mind that trying to do everything at once may force you to stop because it can cause health problems. Here are a few tips for starting and sticking to an exercise regimen:

- Make a plan and respect it.
- Ask your friends and family if they want to go along with you. Mutual motivation will help you to keep it up.
- Do not concentrate on a single activity. Try activities that focus on different parts of your body to vary your daily efforts and keep exercise interesting.
- Give yourself rewards. At the end of each month's exercise, reward yourself with gifts, records, new books, and things that will help you stick with the program.

DASH Diet Exercises

Researchers have provided evidence that weight control increases the cardiovascular benefits obtained from following the DASH Diet. This emphasizes how important it is that you integrate weight loss and exercise into any program that includes changing the lifestyle of people with high blood pressure.

DIFFERENT TYPES OF EXERCISE

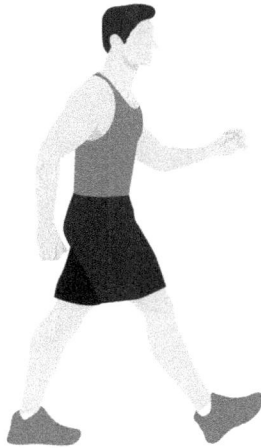

1. Walking

One of the most efficient exercises for burning calories is walking. This is a basic exercise that is extremely easy and requires no special training before implementing it into your routine. Walking can be done almost anywhere, even walking the dog counts. The duration of the walk varies from person to person, but at least thirty minutes per day is recommended. Some people already do this without real-izing it. One way to walk more often is to try using the stairs instead of elevators or escalators whenever possible in your everyday life. Another option is to go places, such as regular errands or shopping downtown, on foot instead of by car.

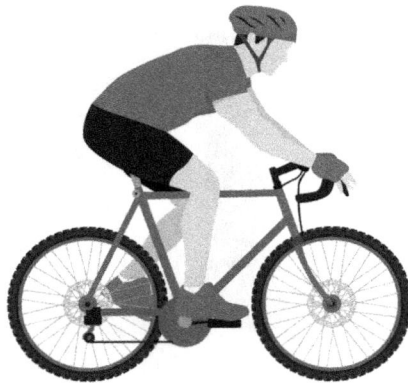

2. Biking

Biking is another great way to easily incorporate cardio into your everyday life. If, for example, the supermarket or your workplace is not close enough to walk to, try biking there instead. Biking is also an efficient and economical form of transport, which will make you feel good and healthy while saving money on gas, parking, or public transit.

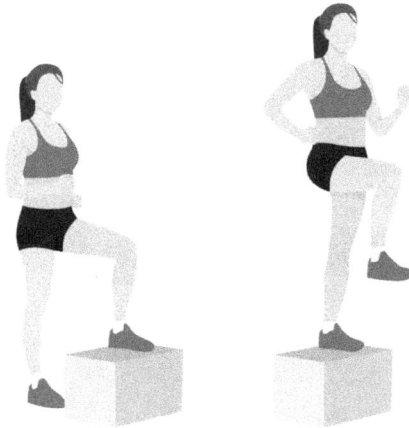

3. Taking the Stairs

As mentioned earlier, taking the stairs instead of the elevator or escalator is an easy way to incorporate more exercise into everyday life. The health benefits of taking the stairs are great: when we take the stairs, we use our upper body and leg muscles, developing strength and improving flexibility. To give an example, climbing ten floors a day (equivalent to walking roughly two and a half miles) will burn an extra 150 calories, compared with taking an elevator. You don't necessarily have to climb all ten floors at once; the effects of taking the stairs are cumulative. You can take two flights at a time, throughout your periodic comings and goings.

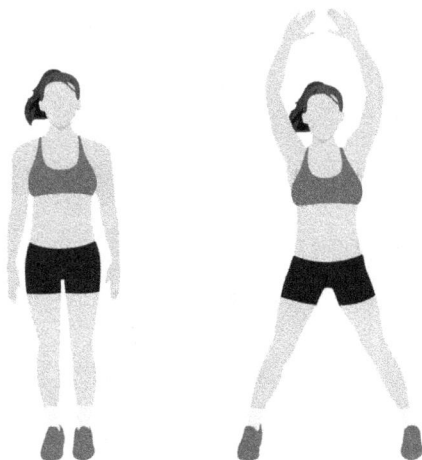

4. Jumping Jacks

Jumping jacks are an exercise often used in the army, also known as New Zealand push-ups. These are often used as a free-body aerobic exercise for an efficient warm-up. Extend your legs and arms, and then jump, gathering your knees toward your chest.

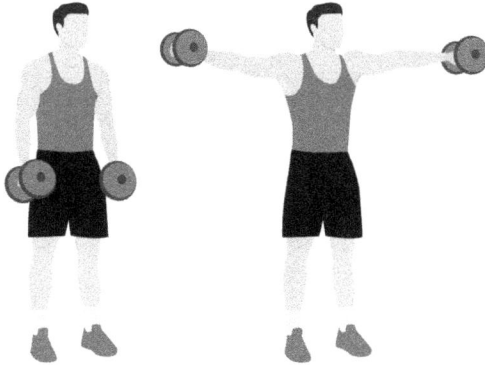

5. Lateral Raise

This exercise is particularly useful for toning the shoulders. Grab light dumbbells (or two half-full bottles of water), start with your hands at your sides, keep your elbows slightly bent, and raise your arms sideways to shoulder level.

The movement must be fluid and soft, and you should not feel any pain. You must perform it smoothly. Repeat 5–7 times, but don't overdo it. You should make changes gradually.

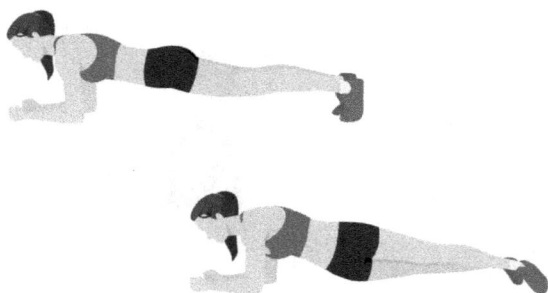

6. Planking

This is one of the best exercises to keep your abdomen strong and stable. Some strength is required, but you can start with a half plank or side plank to gradually build up your strength. To begin, lie down on the floor facing down and lean on your forearms. At this first stage, you are resting and your feet are lying on the ground. Next, use your lower limbs and raise the pelvis so that your back is completely straight. Maintain the position for 30–60 seconds by contracting your abdominal muscles, and then repeat at least five times.

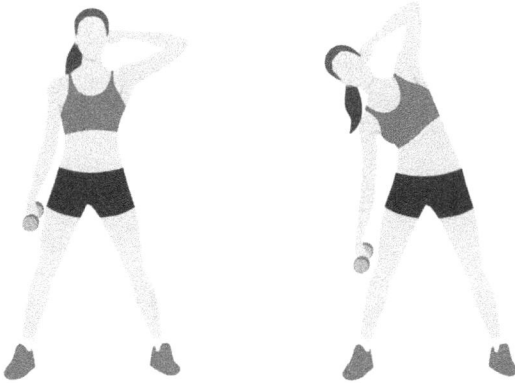

7. Side Bend

This is an exercise for our side abdominal muscles. These muscles are located in the oblique area of the body, and like the diagonal abdominal muscles, they are a little more difficult to train.

The exercise begins with a split jump, in which you move your legs diagonally forward and cross one leg in front of the other. You follow this move by flexing backward so that you return to your original position. In this way, your feet swap positions when moving forward and backward.

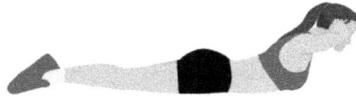

8. Back Extension

Tone and firm your buttock muscles with this exercise. Lie with your stomach on the floor, facing down. Rest your hands on your head, and push with your lower back to lift your chest a few inches from the floor. Return to your starting position, wait about twenty seconds, and then repeat the exercise.

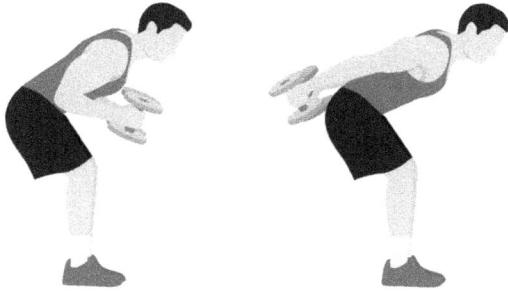

9. Kickbacks

This exercise is particularly helpful for toning of triceps, which are located on the backside of the arm (behind the biceps). To do a kickback, bend forward with your back straight and your abs well stretched (like in a judo greeting). Start with light weights and bent elbows, pointing your hands backward to engage the triceps, and straighten your elbows.

7

THE DASH DIET LIFESTYLE

High blood pressure or hypertension is a pathological condition where the force of blood in your arteries is higher than the normal range. The normal range of systolic blood pressure is 120/80 mmHg, while the normal range for diastolic blood pressure is 90/60 mmHg.

Sometimes, blood pressure can spike due to trauma or an event. These non-consistent spikes are not a diagnosis of hypertension, and the prognosis is not that of someone with diagnosed hypertension. Hypertension is diagnosed when blood pressure consistently measures as a systolic blood pressure of over 130 mmHg and a diastolic blood pressure of over 80 mmHg. Due to the high stress of modern workplaces, an estimated 1.13 billion people have been diagnosed with hypertension, putting them at higher risk of certain fatal health abnormalities. From a dietitian's perspective, the chemical element to look for in diet plans and avoid in any food intake is sodium.

Biologically, sodium increases the volume of plasma in the bloodstream. This, in turn, increases the stroke volume, which then increases the systolic blood pressure in the body; hence, sodium intake is related to increased blood pressure. We live at a time when diet choices are the worst they have ever been. The modern workload favors quick meals, irrespective of their sodium content and health repercussions. Fast-food chains exist in every city, providing customers with quick service and great taste.

The sodium content in fast food is ridiculously high, and the nutrient efficiency is compromised with deep-frying and overcooking. If you are under constant stress and frequently consume fast food with high sodium levels, you are at a much higher risk of developing health irregularities than most people. Obesity is highly correlated with a high risk of hypertension.

Obese patients are also at risk of developing insulin and leptin resistance, which are directly related to hypertension. In addition, obese patients with hypertension are also at a higher risk of multiple health disorders including diabetes, muscular injuries, coronary heart disease, osteoarthritis, and even death.

Today we face an obesity epidemic with most obese patients diagnosed with high blood pressure. Hypertension can be fatal. Fast food contains an absurd amount of sodium. Fast food chains also offer desserts and foods high in sugar content, leading to further obesity and hypertension. Evolutionarily, we are not built to consume so many simple carbohydrates (sugars) as fuel.

Eating sweets in excess spikes blood sugar levels. Blood sugar spikes stimulate the pancreas to make large amounts of insulin, a lot of which is unnecessary; this excess insulin gives you a sugar craving even after you've eaten sweet treats. It's a vicious cycle, and getting out of it takes self-discipline. Recent studies have shown that quitting sugar creates a similar brain response as quitting certain drugs. Sugar can be addictive. Excess sugar is directly related to De Novo lipogenesis, which in non-medical terms, is the process of making fat from non-fat sources. Excess sugar is changed to fat, leading to obesity and hypertension. The pop culture saying that "a moment on the lips is forever on the hips," is actually a reference to the production of fat from sugar. A lifestyle choice of regular exercise will improve your cardiovascular health, control obesity, and keep hypertension under control. Mayo Clinic, a leading medical resource, suggests intense activity of at least thirty minutes per day for good cardiovascular health.

Good cardiovascular health means a healthy pumping heart, which is an integral part of controlling hypertension. Being active, working out, and keeping your body fat percentage within the normal healthy range also help to bring down your insulin levels, increase cell insulin absorption, and lower your risk of developing numerous diseases, including hypertension.

Another high-sodium component of our diet today is fizzy drinks and sodas. Sodas contain high sodium levels and could prove fatal for someone with diagnosed hypertension. Diet drinks eliminate the many sugars that normal drinks contain, but they contain almost five times as much sodium as a normal drink. It is, therefore, better to avoid them altogether. For example, according to the Google calorie counter, 100 grams of Coke contains 5 mg of sodium, but 100 grams of Diet Coke contains 40 mg of sodium.

Because many of the foods you eat at restaurants or that you purchase prepackaged are higher in sodium, how can you incorporate the diet into your day-to-day routine, while still enjoying some of your favorite foods and visiting your favorite establishments to dine out with friends and family?

WHAT TO AVOID

There are some foods you should avoid completely since they are known to cause hypertension. Many of them you may consume without even realizing it. In this section, I will introduce you to some foods that are not meant for people with high blood pressure.

DASH DIET FOR BEGINNERS | 169

- **White bread (made using refined flour).** White bread contains large amounts of refined flour which is not good for your heart. When you consume large quantities of refined flour, you increase your chances of contracting diabetes and coronary heart disease. Still, you may unwittingly consume refined flour. Most foods (such as cakes, biscuits, cookies, etc.) made with refined flour are white in color. If you want to consume bread, it is advisable to choose bread made from unrefined flour, which is brown in color.
- **Canned foods.** Canned foods are very high in sodium. If you want to include canned foods in your diet, then you must read the nutrition information clearly and make sure that they are reduced- or low-sodium options. You may assume that canned foods are healthy and think that you are doing yourself a favor by eating them. Most of the sodium is actually consumed through canned foods.
- **Pasta.** Pasta is very high in salt. Pasta would be very good for your heart if it weren't for the salt. Therefore, if you have hypertension or you're at risk of developing hypertension, you shouldn't eat pasta. If you want to consume pasta, try to choose a whole wheat or low-sodium variety.
- **Snacks, such as chips and some varieties of cheese.** Stay away from snacks and various categories of cheese that are high in sodium. Besides their high

sodium levels, they offer no nutritional value and contain lots of calories. A great example of high-sodium cheese is processed cheese, which contains around 1,000 milligrams of sodium per 100 grams. The four-cheese pizza at restaurants is also very high in sodium. This pizza with no toppings contains around 400 milligrams of sodium. The amount of sodium increases with each topping, so avoid eating these pizzas.

- **Frozen fish or chicken sticks.** Frozen fish and chicken sticks should be avoided as much as possible. First and foremost, these products contain large amounts of sodium since they are mostly preserved with salt. Secondly, these products may contain harmful chemicals from the preservation process. Moreover, frozen fish and chicken sticks are low in nutritional value and there are many suitable alternatives.
- **Frozen meat and dinners.** Frozen meat is also high in salt content. A great example of this is a frozen dinner, which contains around 600 milligrams of sodium per 100 grams.
- **Prebaked and prepackaged cookies.** Prebaked and prepackaged cookies contain large amounts of sodium. They do not actually contain a high number of calories, but they are high in salt, so don't eat too many of these products.

- **Prepackaged cakes and cake mixes.** People often think that packaged cakes and cake mixes make a great addition to their diet when actually many of them don't. In fact, these items are very high in sodium and fat and should be avoided at all costs.
- **Processed meats.** One must stay away from processed meats, especially those preserved with sodium. They are high in both salt and fat. For example, one serving of hot dogs contains around 80 grams of fat and approximately 110 milligrams of sodium.
- **Meal mixes (boxed).** Mixing food ingredients together and storing them in one box is also not good for your health. These often contain high amounts of salt, for preservation and shelf storage. They also rarely have much nutritional content. Therefore, this particular type of food must be avoided as much as possible.
- **Some breakfast cereals.** Certain breakfast cereals are high in preservatives and sugar. They can also be high in sodium content for shelf storage and preservation. You should avoid consuming these types of cereals altogether since they contain a lot of sodium and have very little nutritional value.

Living a healthy lifestyle is quite easy if you know which foods to consume and which to avoid. The idea behind the

DASH Diet is to get all of the nutrients that humans need without eating large amounts of sodium and fat, both of which are harmful in the long run.

8

TIPS ON STICKING WITH YOUR DASH DIET

Change is difficult. Especially if your goal is to develop lifelong healthy habits. You will need encouragement, advice, and planning to help you get through the inevitable rough spots along the way. From navigating the grocery store to dealing with social circumstances, here are a few tips to help you attain DASH Diet success.

You can't start on a new path without knowing where you have been, or you run the risk of backtracking. The best way to begin the DASH Diet, or any new eating plan, is to take an honest look at your current eating habits. Use a food journal and record everything you eat and drink for several days. Take the record one step further and analyze vital nutritional content, including sodium intake. This will give you a clear look at how you must modify your current eating habits to line up with DASH guidelines.

Don't do everything at once. Major changes take time, and if you keep this in mind, you are more likely to be successful with your new dietary lifestyle. Begin by making one or two small changes, and keep with them until they feel natural, before making more changes. For example, switch to low-fat dairy this week and work on adding more produce next week. Gradually increase servings of fresh fruit and vegetables by adding one serving to one meal each day. These gradual changes will be good for your mental commitment and will help your body adjust to the increased fiber and slight detoxification brought about by the elimination of processed foods and excess sodium.

Familiarize yourself with portion sizes. You'll learn that one serving of meat is three to four ounces and that you need to consume four to five servings of vegetables. Still, do you really understand what that looks like and whether eating that amount of food will satisfy you? Understanding what portion sizes look and feel like will go a long way in helping you follow DASH Diet guidelines.

Don't be afraid to ask questions when you dine out or enjoy dinners and parties at a friend's house. Ask how the food was prepared and what ingredients they contain. If you plan on following the DASH Diet for life, there will likely be an occasion here or there where you just let the plan slide. However, if you live a lifestyle where you frequently entertain or eat out, you'll have to step up and ask these questions to eliminate the risk of sabotaging your diet. If you are not comfortable letting your host know of your dietary restrictions, then offer to bring a dish or two to pass around. This will ensure that you also have something to enjoy and do not inconvenience anyone.

Beware of condiments and sauces, as these are often heavy in salt, sugar, and fats. Even the most unassuming ones—such as ketchup—can add milligrams of salt and unwanted sugar to your diet. Ask for foods to be prepared without extra sauces or have them served on the side so that you are in charge of how much you eat.

Accept that you are human. This nutritional plan could be the start of a lifelong approach to healthy eating and wellness protection, as long as you are realistic about your expectations. The plan leaves room for moderation. The main focus should not be on sacrifice, but on making healthy choices most of the time. Allow yourself an occasional treat, your mind and body will both thank you for it.

If your finances allow, invest in some good quality cookware and kitchen utensils. The right cookware will make preparing meals easier and less messy, and the food will taste better. Think about getting nonstick cookware, vegetable steamers, and rice cookers, which eliminate the need for excess cooking oils and ensure effortless preparation. Also, consider investing in good quality spice mills for all of the flavorful and exotic new spices you will experiment with as you change your priorities from salty to flavourful.

Always read labels. *Always.* Pay particular attention to saturated fat, sodium, and fiber content. When something appears high in sodium or fats, weigh what you will give up against what you gain from one portion of that food and ask yourself if it is worth it. In some cases, you may feel that it is. In others, the idea of giving up several servings of other foods will persuade you to put it down and move on to something else.

Don't be afraid to modify your recipes. The DASH Diet isn't about putting your favorites away forever; it is about modifying them so that you can still enjoy them whenever you want to without worrying that you are damaging your health. Make low-fat substitutions, reduce the amount of meat, increase the number of grains or vegetables, and reduce the amount of sugar and salt. For instance, add sugar-free applesauce to reduce the sugar in a muffin recipe, or introduce a nice spice blend to help you forget that you hardly used any salt in your treasured stew recipe.

There should always be something green on your plate, and there should be a lot of it. There is a reason that eating a salad in one meal is not a part of the DASH approach, and that accomplishment requires you to eat more vegetables in the remainder of your meal. When you prepare healthy meals in general, enjoy them; savor the flavors and the textures.

Always judge a recipe by its ingredients, not by its serving size or quantity. This way you will ensure that you maintain the nutrients from each serving when you make adjustments for taste or cost per serving.

Be sure to keep a notebook of what you plan to eat for each week, and make a record of how you felt as you were going through your specific diet plan. By keeping track of your experience following the DASH Diet, you can see how it affects your body and mind. If you feel run-down, tired, or unfocused from not eating enough fiber or certain foods that are now off-limits for a time, then adjust accordingly.

Look for new ways to prepare food. If you love fried food, you could try oven-frying the food using olive oil and whole wheat bread. Consider using low-sodium broth instead of heavy oils for sautéing and learn how to steam, bake, and sauté your favorite foods. The preparation is not only healthier; it's easy and requires little cleanup.

Never allow yourself to go hungry because when you are hungry you are more likely to indulge in the very foods you are trying to cut out of your life. If you find that you are hungry immediately after a meal, then your portions are too small, and you should bulk up your meals a little bit. Keep plenty of fresh healthy snacks available to help curb hunger between meals and drink plenty of water. Make sure to get in at least eight to ten glasses per day.

Never go to the grocery store hungry. Either do your grocery shopping after a meal or keep a healthy snack (such as fruit or vegetables) in your car to nibble on before you go in. If you are not hungry, you are more likely to stick with your dietary plan rather than splurge on things that provide you with no nutrition and too much salt and fat.

Discover the art of meal planning. There are two schools of thought on meal planning: Some people love it and enjoy devoting time to it. Others think it is just too much work and never works out anyway. I am here to tell you that there actually is a happy medium between these two. Even if you are not a fan of meal planning, start by planning half of your meals, even if it is just breakfast or lunch. Write out a menu and what ingredients you need. Maybe a weekly meal plan for breakfast will only include oatmeal, eggs, low-fat yogurt, fresh berries, and asparagus. But you will know each day what you will have, which will help you commit to actually giving yourself time for preparation. You will also know that you have everything you need for each of those meals. Start small and build on it. Soon, you will find that meal planning not only makes grocery shopping easier and is gentler on the wallet, but you will begin to look forward to certain meals throughout the week. This will also help you stay on track with your diet. If you are unsure of where to start with meal planning, there are several apps and websites that are helpful in creating simple weekly meal plans.

Be careful with your condiment choices. For instance, if you choose to put ketchup on your hamburger, ask yourself how it will fit into your healthy diet plan. If not, take it off the burger and see how you like it without ketchup. Add sliced fruit to your cereal or oatmeal for breakfast, instead of fat-laden fruit-flavored syrups. There are many healthier alternatives to traditional condiments. Just make sure that they won't prevent you from achieving your goals.

Choose fresh whenever possible. When fresh produce is an option, choose it over canned. Frozen produce is also an excellent option since they don't contain as much sodium as canned goods. Speaking of frozen foods, limit your choices to frozen vegetables and fruit, avoiding frozen prepared meals and snacks. If you do choose canned goods, rinse off the contents whenever possible. This applies especially to canned vegetables and meats. You can also make your own sauces, salad dressings, and soups to ensure that your food contains natural, fresh ingredients. There is a healthy alternative to just about everything, so you don't have to depend on the frozen food section for your favorite snacks or meals.

Learn to shop the perimeter of the store. This is where you will find the foods that are promoted on the DASH Diet plan. Along the perimeter or outside aisles of your grocery store, you will find fresh produce, dairy, meat, seafood and possibly a bakery where you can purchase fresh whole-grain bread. Save the middle aisles for things such as additional grains and spices only. Flavor isn't just about the spice aisle. Yes, I've repeatedly made the point about choosing other spices over salt, but you should also consider other foods that add incredible flavor to your dishes, like onion, garlic, fresh ginger, citrus, vinegar, and low-sodium sauces.

Try cooking without meat at least twice a week. Although this isn't a necessity, it is a good way to build up your repertoire of healthier recipes and reduce your sodium intake. Even if you aren't a vegetarian, meatless dinners can offer a great change of pace and help you continue making healthier eating decisions.

Have a support system. Even better, have a multilevel support system. Get your family and friends involved in your decision and ask someone to be your accountability partner. These are the people that you will go to when you have difficulty sticking to the plan. We all start out with pure intentions, but when we are honest with ourselves; we know there will be times when we need a little nudge to stay on track. This is what your support is for. It is helpful to have a medical support system that includes a physician or dietician that can help you along the way as you encounter questions or require evaluation.

Finally, reward yourself for a job well done, and forgive yourself when things don't go as planned. What are the things you dreamed about doing or accomplishing when you become healthier or lose some weight? Was it a new outfit, the confidence to finally join that group fitness class, run a half marathon, or take that spa trip with friends that you always found a way to talk yourself out of? These are the things you should reward yourself with as you reach your personal goals. But also, be gentle with yourself. You are setting out on a new road, and along the way, there will be bumps, and you may feel shaken enough to leave the path. You are more likely to stay true to your goals when you allow yourself to make a few mistakes. Changing your lifestyle is a long-term process, and it is an ongoing learning adventure. When you slip up, evaluate the cause and learn from your mistake. Forgive yourself, dust yourself off, and carry on. This is the path to success.

Tips for Lowering Your Salt Intake

Over time, sodium has become just as pervasive as fat and sugar. Consuming excessive amounts of sodium can lead to high blood pressure, diabetes, kidney disease, and muscle cramps.

The following steps can help to lower your sodium intake:

- Take the salt shaker off the table.
- Season your food using herbs and spices instead of salt. This is the best way to enhance the flavor without adding more salt.
- Always rinse your vegetables before you eat them.
- Opt for the lower sodium versions of the food you love most.
- Check canned, frozen, and prepared foods for sodium content. The Food and Drug Administration (FDA) has strict regulations regarding the labeling of sodium on processed foods. The sodium content appears on the top half of the nutrition facts label.

Avoid those with a high sodium content and choose foods with a salt content of less than 5 percent of the daily value.

Vitamins and Minerals to Help with Lowering Your Sodium Intake

Below are some vitamins and minerals that can help with sodium reduction in your diet:

1. Vitamin B6

This vitamin works with many of our bodies' enzymes. It is involved in protein metabolism and blood glucose regulation. B6 encourages the use of glucose for energy through glycogenesis. B6 also metabolizes iron and allows for adequate absorption of iron from food sources. Additionally, B6 helps to reduce fatigue and stress-related fatigue, and it enhances fatty acid utilization. The recommended daily amount of Vitamin B6 is 1.3 milligrams per day.

2. Magnesium

This mineral not only helps our bodies to detox but also helps us to maintain electrolyte balance in our body fluids. Magnesium is critical for the production of ATP, which helps with muscle contraction and relaxation. Additionally, magnesium is responsible for bone growth and develop-

DASH DIET FOR BEGINNERS | 183

ment. The recommended daily amount of magnesium ranges from 310 to 320 milligrams per day.

3. Calcium

This mineral is essential for our bone health. It is also a critical component of muscles and nerves. Calcium assists with blood clotting, nerve function, and hormone secretion. The recommended daily amount of calcium ranges from 1,000 to 1,300 milligrams per day.

4. Potassium

This mineral increases muscle contractions and helps with the maintenance of the body's fluid balance. Potassium is also involved in metabolism, nerve impulse transmission, and enzyme function. The recommended daily amount of potassium ranges from 2,000 to 2,500 milligrams per day.

5. Vitamin C

Vitamin C is essential for immunity, the repair of injured tissues, and the formation of collagen. The recommended daily amount of Vitamin C ranges from 120 to 160 milligrams per day.

6. Vitamin D

Vitamin D is essential for calcium absorption, bone metabolism, and immune response to infections. The recommended daily amount of Vitamin D ranges from 600 to 800 IU per day.

7. Vitamin E

This vitamin improves circulation, maintains blood vessel walls, and helps to break down cholesterol. The recommended daily amount ranges from 10 mg to 15 mg per day.

FINAL WORDS

The DASH Diet is a well-known, functional, and healthful eating plan. It's a well-balanced diet that covers all dietary groups. The human body is made of various chemical components necessary for good health. This nutritional plan aims to provide the body with all the essential nutrients. It restricts only unhealthy food choices to avoid raising blood pressure and developing hypertension. Hypertension is linked to several health complications like stroke, cardiovascular diseases, and other health issues. Adopting a healthy eating pattern like the DASH Diet can significantly reduce the risk of these complications and improve the overall quality of life.

This diet is characterized by the consumption of various fruits, vegetables, nuts, legumes, and low-fat dairy products. It has a huge impact on an individual's blood pressure, total cholesterol, and blood glucose levels. To follow the DASH Diet, you must limit your sodium intake to 2,300 milligrams per day. The typical American diet is very unhealthy and includes a lot of processed and sugar-sweetened foods. These food products also have a very high sodium content, exceeding daily recommendations. In this regard, limiting sodium levels is an effective way to reduce the level of hypertension. This diet was developed for managing hypertension, but researchers have proven that it can help with weight loss and can help to avoid other health diseases. Healthy eating leads to healthy living, and the DASH Diet is the best choice to fight against chronic diseases. It also has many environmental benefits. People can enjoy delicious food on this diet.

This diet also has some downsides. People on a DASH Diet for an extended period can face kidney problems because of high potassium, magnesium, and calcium levels. Another drawback is bloating due to the high fiber. A dietician can help to eliminate these downsides. The DASH Diet is effective for diabetic patients or those diagnosed with heart disease. Different types of foods play an integral part in this diet. The DASH Diet is an all-around good choice for health, but you should always consult your doctor or dietitian when making dietary changes. It's also important to continue regular exercise when on this nutritional plan.

At first look, some low-fat diets may appear to be an excellent option for losing weight and lowering blood pressure.

They can, however, put people with certain health issues, such as high blood pressure, in danger. The DASH Diet is considered a safe and effective strategy for reducing weight and keeping sodium levels low.

Now that you have all the tools, go out there and make the DASH Diet work for you! Remember, this diet is a lifestyle choice and not a traditional fad "diet." Do what works for you to obtain your health goals, and be patient along the way.

REFERENCES

Blumenthal, J. A., Babyak, M. A., Hinderliter, A., Watkins, L. L., Craighead, L., Lin, P. H., ... & Sherwood, A. (2010). "Effects of the DASH diet alone and in combination with exercise and weight loss on blood pressure and cardio-vascular biomarkers in men and women with high blood pressure: The ENCORE study." *Archives of Internal Medicine*, 170(2), 126–135.

Chatham, J. (2012). *The DASH Diet Health Plan: Low-Sodium, Low-Fat Recipes to Promote Weight Loss, Lower Blood Pressure and Help Prevent Diabetes.* Callisto Media, Inc.

Chatham, J. (2013). *The DASH Diet for Beginners: Essentials to Get Started.* Callisto Media, Inc.

Moore, L. L., Bradlee, M. L., Singer, M. R., Qureshi, M. M., Buendia, J. R., & Daniels, S. R. (2012). "Dietary Approaches to Stop Hypertension (DASH) eating pattern and risk of elevated blood pressure in adolescent girls." *British Journal of Nutrition*, 108(9), 1678–1685.

Most, M. M. (2004). "Estimated phytochemical content of the dietary approaches to stop hypertension (DASH) diet is higher than in the Control Study Diet." *Journal of the American Dietetic Association*, 104(11), 1725--1727.

Nishat, F. (2020). "Meal Preparation Strategies and Dietary Information to Help Prevent Recurrent Stroke."

Press, S. (2013). *The DASH Diet for Beginners: The Guide to Getting Started.* Arcas Publishing.

Press, T. (2014). *The DASH Diet for Every Day: 4 Weeks of DASH Diet Recipes & Meal Plans to Lose Weight & Improve Health.* Callisto Media, Inc.

Razavi Zade, M., Telkabadi, M. H., Bahmani, F., Salehi, B., Farshbaf, S., & Asemi, Z. (2016). "The effects of DASH diet on weight loss and metabolic status in adults with non-alcoholic fatty liver disease: A randomized clinical trial." *Liver International*, 36(4), 563–571.

Rozewicki, J., Li, S., Amada, K. M., Standley, D. M., & Katoh, K. (2019). "MAFFT-DASH: Integrated protein sequence and structural alignment." *Nucleic Acids Research*, 47(W1), W5–W10.

Ryan, D. H., & Champagne, C. (2003). "Better nutrient data improves public health: Evidence and examples from the Dietary Approaches to Stop Hypertension (DASH) Trial." *Journal of Food Composition and Analysis*, 16(3), 313–321.

Sacks, F. M., Svetkey, L. P., Vollmer, W. M., Appel, L. J., Bray, G. A., Harsha, D., ... & Cutler, J. A. (2001). "Effects on blood pressure of reduced dietary sodium and the Dietary Approaches to Stop Hypertension (DASH) diet." *New England Journal of Medicine*, 344(1), 3–10.

Alessa, T., Hawley, M., Hock, E., and de Witte, L.D. (2019). "Smartphone apps to support self-management of hypertension: Review and content analysis." *JMIR mHealth and uHealth*, 7. n. pag. https://www.semanticscholar.org/paper/Smartphone-Apps-to-Support-Self-Management-of-and-Alessa-Hawley/b0c9dffabababdc819476144fe2a112038ff732c?p2df.

Steinberg, D., Bennett, G. G., & Svetkey, L. (2017). "The DASH diet, 20 years later." *Jama*, 317(15), 1529–1530.

Svetkey, L. P., Simons-Morton, D. G., Proschan, M. A., Sacks, F. M., Conlin, P. R., Harsha, D., ... & DASH-Sodium Collaborative Research Group. (2004). "Effect of the dietary approaches to stop hypertension diet and reduced sodium intake on blood pressure control." *The Journal of Clinical Hypertension*, 6(7), 373–381.

Svetkey, L. P., Simons-Morton, D., Vollmer, W. M., Appel, L. J., Conlin, P. R., Ryan, D. H., ... & DASH Research Group. (1999). "Effects of dietary patterns on blood pressure: subgroup analysis of the Dietary Approaches to Stop Hypertension (DASH) randomized clinical trial." *Archives of Internal Medicine*, 159(3), 285–293.

Van den Brink, A. C., Brouwer-Brolsma, E. M., Berendsen, A. A., & van de Rest, O. (2019). "The Mediterranean, Dietary Approaches to Stop Hypertension (DASH), and Mediterranean-DASH Intervention for Neurodegenerative Delay (MIND) diets are associated with less cognitive decline and a lower risk of Alzheimer's disease—a review." *Advances in Nutrition*, 10(6), 1040–1065.

Yao, Y., Chen, S. B., Ding, G., & Dai, J. (2019). "Evaluation of Reliability of the Recomputed Nutrient Intake Data in the National Heart, Lung, and Blood Institute Twin Study." *Nutrients*, 11(1), 109.

www.ingramcontent.com/pod-product-compliance
Lightning Source LLC
Chambersburg PA
CBHW032056020426
42335CB00011B/362